FRAMEWORKS FOR
RADIOLOGY REPORTING

DEDICATION

To my wife, Amanda, who through her good humour and unending support has made me realize there are far more important things in life than radiology.

JJ

In loving memory of my uncle, Dr C. Bhuvaneswaran, Associate Professor of Biochemistry, University of Arkansas, who first inspired me to pursue a career in medicine.

And finally, Mavis Grace, will you marry me?

RA

FRAMEWORKS FOR RADIOLOGY REPORTING

Edited by

Joseph Jacoby

BSc MBBS MRCP

Specialist Registrar in Radiology,
Southampton General Hospital,
Southampton, UK

Ravi Ayer

BSc MB MRCS

Specialist Registrar in Radiology,
Southampton General Hospital,
Southampton, UK

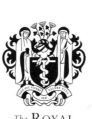

The ROYAL
SOCIETY *of*
MEDICINE
PRESS *Limited*

Published by the Royal Society of Medicine Press Ltd
1 Wimpole Street, London W1G 0AE, UK
Tel: +44 (0)20 7290 2921
Fax: +44 (0)20 7290 2929
Email: publishing@rsm.ac.uk
Website: www.rsmpress.co.uk

British Library Cataloguing in Publication Data
A catalogue record for this book is available from the British Library

ISBN 978-1-85315-820-9

Distribution in Europe and Rest of World:

Marston Book Services Ltd
PO Box 269
Abingdon
Oxon OX14 4YN, UK
Tel: +44 (0)1235 465500
Fax: +44 (0)1235 465555
Email: direct.order@marston.co.uk

Distribution in the USA and Canada:

Royal Society of Medicine Press Ltd
c/o BookMasters Inc
30 Amberwood Parkway
Ashland, OH 44805, USA
Tel: +1 800 247 6553/+1 800 266 5564
Fax: +1 419 281 6883
Email: order@bookmasters.com

Distribution in Australia and New Zealand:

Elsevier Australia
30-52 Smidmore Street
Marrickville NSW 2204, Australia
Tel: +61 2 9517 8999
Fax: +61 2 9517 2249
Email: service@elsevier.com.au

Typeset by Phoenix Photosetting, Chatham, Kent
Printed in the UK by Bell & Bain, Glasgow

CONTENTS

CONTRIBUTING AUTHORS

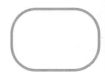

Ravi Ayer BSc MB MRCS
Specialist Registrar in Radiology, Southampton General Hospital, Southampton, UK

Vincent Batty BSc MBBS DMRD FRCR MSc
Consultant in Radiology and Nuclear Medicine, Southampton University Hospitals NHS Trust, Southampton, UK

Richard Blaquiere BSc MBChB FRCR
Consultant Radiologist, Southampton University Hospitals NHS Trust, Southampton, UK

Keith Dewbury BSc MBBS DMRD FRCR
Consultant Radiologist and Honorary Senior Lecturer, Southampton University Hospitals NHS Trust, Southampton, UK

Joanna Fairhurst MBBS MA MRCP FRCR
Consultant in Paediatric Radiology, Southampton University Hospitals NHS Trust, Southampton, UK

Stephen Harden MA MBBS FRCS FRCR
Consultant in Cardiothoracic Radiology, Southampton University Hospitals NHS Trust, Southampton, UK

Joseph Jacoby BSc MBBS MRCP
Specialist Registrar in Radiology, Southampton General Hospital, Southampton, UK

Jason MacDonald MBBS MRCP FRCR
Fellow in Neuroradiology, Royal Prince Alfred Hospital, Sydney, Australia

Caroline Rubin MBBS MRCP FRCR
Consultant Radiologist, Southampton University Hospitals NHS Trust, Southampton, UK

Madeleine Sampson MBChB MRCP FRCR
Consultant in Musculoskeletal Radiology, Southampton University Hospitals NHS Trust, Southampton, UK

Francis Sundram MBChB BAO Bmed BSc MRCP(Ireland) MRCPS(Glasgow) MSc
Consultant in Nuclear Medicine, Southampton University Hospitals NHS Trust,
Southampton, UK

David Thompson MBBS FRCS FRCP
Consultant in Vascular Interventional Radiology, Southampton University Hospitals
NHS Trust, Southampton, UK

ACKNOWLEDGEMENTS

We are extremely grateful to all the contributors who gave up their valuable time to help us over the last year. We would particularly like to thank Caroline Rubin and Madeleine Sampson, who dedicated a disproportionately large amount of time to this book. We would also like to thank Sarah Ogden, Sarah Vasey and Hannah Wessely at RSM Press for all their advice and assistance. Finally, we would like to thank Stephen Harden, whose reporting ethos and teaching style inspired us to write this book in the first place.

FOREWORD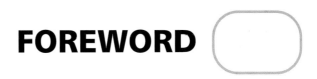

The most important step in treating the patient is making the diagnosis, and imaging continues to assume an increasingly important role in this respect.

Image analysis, and ultimately the construction of the formal report, is often learnt by a process of osmosis. Based on their own experience, as they have progressed through their training, the authors have written a text that will help the inexperienced develop a logical, systematic approach to image analysis at an early stage in their training.

There is no substitute for experience, but I have no doubt this excellent text will be an invaluable framework on which to build and modify reporting skills.

The best ideas are often the simplest. It is perhaps surprising that this topic has not been addressed in this way before. I have no doubt that this timely text will fulfil a valuable role for the radiology trainee.

Keith Dewbury BSc MBBS DMRD FRCR
Consultant Radiologist and Honorary Senior Lecturer,
Southampton University Hospitals NHS Trust, Southampton, UK

PREFACE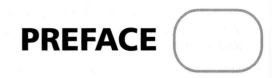

When reporting an image, it is important to draw the findings together in a coherent, coordinated way in order to reach a diagnosis. It is critical not to make random, disconnected observations. One way to avoid this pitfall is to adopt a systematic approach to film viewing.

It is commonly agreed that a logical, systematic approach to image interpretation is advantageous. It ensures that as much information as possible is extracted from the image, whether directly related or incidental to the original indication. Adopting a systematic approach, a reproducible framework for image interpretation, will give you confidence.

Radiologists develop their own individual systems for reporting over many years, based on personal experience. These systems are largely problem based, that is, the analysis is directed at identifying a cause for the presentation. However, if systems were solely problem based, then important peripheral information or incidental diagnoses would be missed. In reality, a combination of both problem-based and general frameworks are used in everyday practice. The general systems outlined here should serve as a good starting point for reporting, before you develop your own approach.

The frameworks outlined in the following pages are intended to assist the trainee radiologist commencing the complex process of image interpretation. They will answer some of the questions that we asked at the beginning of our training, such as:

❑ Where do I start?
❑ What common pathologies should I expect to encounter?
❑ On which projection/window/sequence do I look?
❑ Have I covered everything?

It is perhaps worth mentioning at this early stage what this book is not:

❑ It is not a shortcut to accurate reporting, as there is no substitute for experience, reading around the subject or the advice handed down from senior colleagues.
❑ It does not outline a system for every conceivable radiological examination. We have chosen to include what we consider the most commonly requested and reported investigations that radiology trainees would be expected to interpret with some degree of competence in the early years of their training.
❑ It is not intended to be a comprehensive pathological or pictorial review. Rather,

it is intended to be an easily accessible reference, to be used in conjunction with other learning resources. We have, however, included selected images to illustrate important points and principles of interpretation.

References have not been included in the text, as the frameworks are intended to be stand-alone, practical guides. However, in a few places we have suggested that you have to hand a guide to normal variants. We would recommend Keats and Anderson's *Atlas of Normal Roentgen Variants That May Simulate Disease* (7th edn, Mosby, 2001). We have also included a list of useful texts as further reading, at the end of the book.

We were motivated to write this book as we feel that it would have been an invaluable resource at the start of our training. We sincerely hope that it will be of help to those embarking on a new career in radiology.

Joseph Jacoby and Ravi Ayer

LIST OF FIGURES AND TABLES

FIGURES

TABLES

ABBREVIATIONS

ACA   anterior cerebral artery
AP   anteroposterior
CC   cranio-caudal
CD   Crohn's disease
CNS   central nervous system
CP   chronic pancreatitis
CSF   cerebrospinal fluid
CT   computed tomography
DVT   deep-vein thrombosis
DWI   diffusion-weighted imaging
ECG   electrocardiogram
ENT   ear, nose, throat
IVC   inferior vena cava
IVU   intravenous urogram
MAA   microaggregates of albumin
MCA   middle cerebral artery
MLO   mediolateral oblique
MRI   magnetic resonance imaging
OM   occipito-mental
OM30   occipito-mental 30°
PA   posteroanterior
PCA   posterior cerebral artery
PD   proton density
PE   pulmonary embolism
SAH   subarachnoid haemorrhage
SBO   small-bowel obstruction
SCC   squamous cell carcinoma
STIR   short-tau inversion recovery
V̇/Q̇   ventilation–perfusion

GENERAL PRINCIPLES OF IMAGE INTERPRETATION AND REPORTING

The role of the radiologist is to offer an informed medical opinion, based on the available images, to facilitate the most appropriate next step in management. The following hints and tips can be applied to any individual reporting episode, and we hope that they will prove useful to anyone beginning the task of image interpretation.

Before you start

❏ Ensure that the conditions are right for reporting. Use good-quality viewing conditions in a quiet environment where you are unlikely to be interrupted.
❏ Make sure that you have adequate views and that the images are technically sound. If the images are not diagnostically adequate, it is better to repeat the investigation than to risk missing an important abnormality.

Supplementary information

❏ When reporting, arm yourself with as much information as possible. Make full use of old imaging results, recent blood tests and clinic letters to inform your report as fully as possible.
❏ Talk to clinicians. If in doubt, ring up the referrer to gain further information, which may aid your interpretation of the images.
❏ Always look at previous imaging. An equivocal lung nodule that has a similar appearance 4 years ago is significantly less clinically relevant than one that was not evident 6 months previously.

During interpretation

❏ Be methodical and systematic in your approach to film viewing. Take the time to analyse each investigation thoroughly. You will learn more by looking at fewer studies in detail than by rushing through as many as possible in one sitting.
❏ If one abnormality is identified, continue to search for additional abnormalities, avoiding the pitfall of 'satisfaction of search'.
❏ Look at the contralateral side for comparison.
❏ Always ask a senior colleague if at all in doubt. However, it is important at least to attempt interpretation of the potential abnormality; it will not serve your educational interests to seek help at the first sign of uncertainty.

Composing the final report

❏ Aim to use the same simple three-part format:
  – Clinical information – including the question posed
  – Findings – the main body of the report
  – Conclusion – directed at answering the question.
  A potential exception to this system is when reporting certain plain film studies, when the body of the report and conclusion may be combined.
❏ Try to lay out the body of the report in a logical way, starting with the salient features first, moving on to incidental findings later.
❏ Although using a systematic approach will help ensure that you cover as much as possible, when composing the final report aim to be concise, and mention only the relevant positive and negative findings.
❏ Avoid simply repeating the body of the report in the conclusion. Try to draw the findings together and answer the question posed in the context of the overall clinical picture.
❏ It is not always possible to answer the clinical question definitively. If doubt remains, it is important to communicate this; however, try to suggest further tests that may help resolve any unanswered questions.

Finally ...

❏ Try not to get downhearted when you miss an abnormality, as this happens to even the best and most experienced radiologists. Learn from your mistakes and try to avoid making the same mistake twice.

NEURORADIOLOGY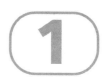

BRAIN CT AND MRI

When reporting brain CT and MR scans, it is important to be aware of the strengths and limitations of each modality. MRI is the superior modality in early infarct diagnosis, defining a tumour and diagnosing subtle collections. CT is better in trauma, with its superior bony definition, and in cases of suspected subarachnoid haemorrhage.

It is important to develop a system for reporting brain CT and MRI scans, one that includes important review areas. Getting to grips with commonly encountered and important pathology is essential. As the approach to reviewing CT and MRI scans is similar, the two are dealt with together below.

Images and sequences

It is vital to appreciate what images and sequences have been acquired. CT images are typically presented as brain and bone algorithms. Note whether intravenous contrast has been given.

Recognizing MRI sequences can initially be difficult, but becomes easier with experience. Start with the conventional sequences in your institution and first become familiar with T1- and T2-weighted sequences.

Previous neurosurgery and hardware

Look at the skull for evidence of previous craniotomy, craniectomy or burr hole. Shunt catheters, drains or reservoirs must be identified and assessed for complications. Aneurysm clips or endovascular coils should be correctly identified. Appreciating previous surgery will make interpreting intracranial findings more straightforward.

Brain parenchyma

The brain parenchyma consists of the cerebral hemispheres, cerebellum and brain stem (midbrain, pons and medulla). Assess these areas for pathology, paying attention to those areas of brain where subtle pathology can have clinically devastating sequelae.

Is there any loss of symmetry?

Interpretation relies heavily on symmetry or the loss of it. Although small degrees of asymmetry are observed in normal cranial anatomy, loss of symmetry should draw the attention of the radiologist. Once identified, the cause should be differentiated between mass effect and volume loss (see 'Signs of mass effect', below).

Is there a loss of grey–white differentiation?

In the normal brain, white matter can be differentiated from the grey matter of the cortex, basal ganglia and thalami. Loss of this definition should be considered abnormal. Distinguishing white from grey matter is easier with MRI than CT. This can be either a localized or a diffuse finding. If localized, suspect infarct; if diffuse, consider cerebral hypoxic injury.

Diffuse hypoxic injury

Diffuse hypoxic injury will usually have a corresponding clinical history. An abnormal CT will typically demonstrate generalized loss of grey–white differentiation, often with diffuse parenchymal low attenuation. A normal CT scan does not exclude this diagnosis and MRI may be useful.

Interpretation Tips

Diffuse hypoxic injury

Grey–white differentiation of the cerebellum may be preserved, producing the 'bright cerebellum' sign. The cerebellar density is actually normal, but appears high relative to the abnormal low-density cerebrum.

Is there evidence of diffuse cerebral swelling?

Normal cerebral convexity sulci and cerebellar fissures should be visible and seen to contain CSF. CSF is also normally identified in the ventricles and basal cisterns.

In diffuse cerebral swelling, the hemispheres expand and efface the convexity sulci, basal cisterns and ventricles. The cerebellum may also be involved. Diffuse swelling may result in uncal herniation and cerebellar tonsillar descent. The cause of the diffuse swelling should be looked for.

Is there a focal abnormality?

Is there high density?

Very high density is usually due to haemorrhage or calcification. Physiological calcification is commonly encountered in the choroid plexus, pineal gland and basal ganglia. Acute haemorrhage is usually associated with a degree of mass effect. Some tumours are slightly hyperdense compared with white matter on unenhanced CT.

Intracerebral haemorrhage

Intracerebral haemorrhage arises from within the brain parenchyma. Hypertension is a common cause, typically in the basal ganglia and deep white matter. Amyloid angiopathy is a common cause in elderly patients.

Interpretation Tips

Intracerebral haemorrhage

● Atypical patterns of intracerebral haemorrhage should raise the suspicion of an underlying tumour, vascular malformation or venous thrombosis. In cases of suspected tumour, follow-up CT at 6–8 weeks may be useful.
● Haemorrhage at specific sites can give clues to the underlying aetiology (Fig. 1.1).
● Be familiar with the changing appearance over time of intracerebral haemorrhage on CT (Table 1.1).
● Be familiar with the changing appearances over time of intracerebral haematoma on MRI (Table 1.2).

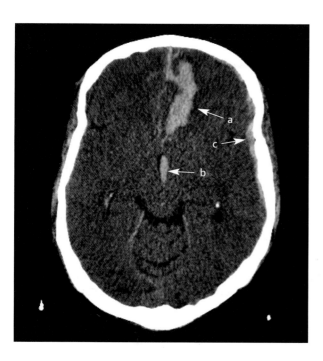

Fig. 1.1. Intracranial haemorrhage. Note high-density blood within the left frontal lobe (a), third ventricle (b) and subdural space (c). Be aware of bleeds around the circle of Willis. The site of the bleed can give an indication as to the cause, in this case a ruptured anterior communicating artery aneurysm.

Is there low density?

Check for areas of low density. Is there an associated mass effect or volume loss? Oedema will typically produce a mass effect. Distinguishing vasogenic (white matter) oedema from cytotoxic oedema is crucial (Table 1.3 and Fig. 1.2).

Table 1.1. The changing appearance over time of haemorrhage on CT

Time from haemorrhage	CT appearances
Hyperacute (<2 hours)	Mixed density (40–60 HU)
Acute (3–48 hours)	High density relative to normal grey matter (60–80 HU)
Early subacute (3–7 days)	Low-density periphery with denser centre
Late subacute (2–4 weeks)	Haematoma density decreases from periphery inwards and may ring enhance, mimicking tumour
Chronic (>1 month)	Density of CSF, typically with loss of volume

Table 1.2. The changing appearance over time of haemorrhage on MRI

Time from haemorrhage	Blood products	T1-weighted signal	T2-weighted signal
Hyperacute (<12 hours)	Oxyhaemoglobin	Isointense	High
Acute (12–72 hours)	Deoxyhaemoglobin	Isointense	Low
Early subacute (4–7 days)	Intracellular methaemoglobin	High	Low
Late subacute (8–30 days)	Extracellular methaemoglobin	High	High
Chronic (>1 month)	Haemosiderin and ferritin	Low	Low

Table 1.3. Distinguishing vasogenic oedema from cytotoxic oedema

	Common causes	Mechanism	CT features
Vasogenic oedema	Tumour abscess	Increased vascular permeability leads to increased extracellular fluid tracking between neuronal axons	Low attenuation involving white matter and sparing cortex
Cytotoxic oedema	Infarct	Cell swelling and death	Low attenuation involving cortex and white matter

Old established infarcts, chronic small-vessel disease and old brain injury (either traumatic or surgical) may also produce cerebral low density. Demyelination may also produce low density on CT; however, MRI is better for imaging demyelinating disease (Fig. 1.3).

In the trauma setting, check the surface of the brain for contusions. Contusions may contain haemorrhage, either acutely or as they mature. Contusions represent direct cerebral trauma and are usually seen where the cortex impacts on the adjacent skull. Typical sites are the inferior frontal and anterior temporal lobes.

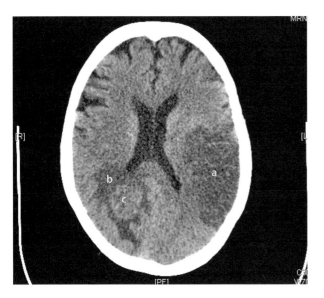

Fig. 1.2. Cytotoxic and vasogenic oedema. This CT scan demonstrates a well-defined area of low attenuation within the left fronto-parietal region secondary to infarction, involving both white and cortical grey matter – cytotoxic oedema (a). The area of low attenuation within the right occipital region spares the cortex – vasogenic oedema (b), in this case due to a glioblastoma (c).

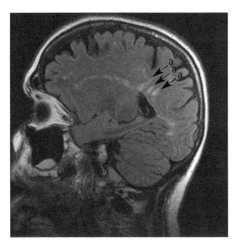

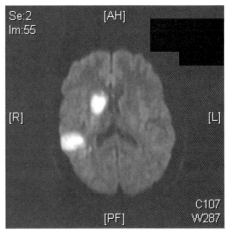

Fig. 1.3. Demyelination may be visualized on CT as patchy low density in the white matter; however, MRI is the superior modality. This sagittal-fluid-suppressed T2-weighted (FLAIR) MRI shows high-signal white-matter lesions orientated perpendicular to the ventricles (a) – the typical appearances of demyelinating plaques of multiple sclerosis.

Fig. 1.4. Hyperacute right-sided MCA territory infarcts on DWI. The corresponding CT was unremarkable.

Infarct

The early CT findings of acute infarction are subtle, but the features become more obvious over time. Early diagnosis is important since the advent of thrombolysis. It is important to assess the middle cerebral artery (MCA), anterior cerebral artery

(ACA), posterior cerebral artery (PCA), perforator and cerebellar vascular territories.

Normal CT does not exclude an acute infarct. MRI is more sensitive to early infarcts, with diffusion-weighted imaging (DWI) providing the earliest detection (Fig. 1.4). Infarcts typically return high signal on T2-weighted and low signal on T1-weighted sequences. The CT findings are summarized in Table 1.4.

Table 1.4. CT findings for infarcts

Acute infarction	Subacute infarction	Old, established infarction
Loss of grey–white differentiation	Cytotoxic oedema in a vascular territory	Parenchymal volume loss
Insular ribbon sign – low attenuation of the insular cortex in early MCA territory infarct	Secondary haemorrhagic transformation	White matter and cortical low attenuation
Lentiform nucleus – occlusion of the lenticulostriate branches of the MCA can lead to obscuration of the lentiform nucleus	Surrounding mass effect	Encephalomalacia with cystic transformation
Dense MCA sign – dense thrombus, typically in proximal MCA or internal carotid artery		
White matter low density		
Subtle mass effect		
No evident abnormality		

MCA, middle cerebral artery.

Interpretation Tips

CT findings for infarcts

● As early infarcts are subtle on CT, it is worth re-reading the clinical information and then reviewing the area of the brain where an infarct is clinically suspected. Fig. 1.5 demonstrates a subtle early infarct.
● In cases with multiple infarcts within a vascular territory, particularly in a younger patient, arterial dissection must be considered.

Masses

Where an intracranial mass is suspected, a systematic appraisal of the clinical and radiological features can narrow the differential diagnosis. Give contrast if a lesion is suspected.

Patient's age

Certain tumours occur more commonly in children than in adults.

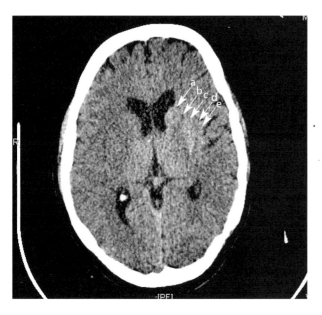

Fig. 1.5. Subtle acute right MCA infarct on CT. Observe the normal left-sided structures – head of caudate (a), internal capsule (b), lentiform nucleus (c), external capsule (d) and insular cortex (e). They are not well seen on the right owing to loss of grey–white differentiation. There is also subtle sulcal effacement on the right.

Solitary or multiple lesions?

Multiple lesions imply a metastatic, infectious or demyelinating aetiology.

Location

It is key to identify whether the lesion is intra-axial (i.e. within the substance of the CNS) or extra-axial (i.e. outside the CNS, but arising from meninges, vessels or other surrounding structures) (Table 1.5).

Table 1.5. Intrà-axial and extra-axial lesions

Intra-axial	Extra-axial
Narrows CSF space	Widens CSF space and may have CSF cleft at its deep border
Cortex displaced peripherally	Cortex and pial vessels displaced away from the skull vault. May cause cortical buckling
Grey–white interface may become ill defined	Grey–white interface typically preserved
May spread across defined anatomical boundaries	May have broad dural base or dural tail with changes in adjacent bone

Whether the lesion is supratentorial or infratentorial may help narrow the differential diagnosis.

Imaging characteristics

Note the density on CT and signal characteristics on MRI.

Is the lesion cystic or solid? If solid, does it contain fat or soft tissue? Does it contain gas? Is there haemorrhage or calcification? This is best assessed with CT.

Contrast enhancement characteristics
Note whether the lesion displays contrast enhancement. Terms such as 'uniform', 'patchy' and 'ring enhancement' may be useful.

Ring enhancement represents the interruption of the blood–brain barrier. The differential diagnosis includes:

- ❏ primary brain tumour
- ❏ metastasis
- ❏ cerebral abscess
- ❏ subacute intracerebral haematoma
- ❏ subacute infarct
- ❏ demyelinating plaque.

Signs of mass effect

Mass effect can be described as distortion of tissue surrounding a lesion, which in turn may produce local or generalized raised intracranial pressure.

Describe how the mass effect distorts normal structures. Note whether there is:

- ❏ effacement of sulci
- ❏ effacement of basal cisterns
- ❏ effacement of the ventricular system (is there secondary hydrocephalus?)
- ❏ midline shift (best assessed by the position of the septum pellucidum)
- ❏ subfalcine herniation
- ❏ uncal (transtentorial) herniation
- ❏ cerebellar tonsillar descent or brain-stem herniation.

Interpretation Tips

Signs of mass effect

- ● Signs of mass effect may be localized. Effacement of a single basal cistern or part of a ventricle may be the only sign of mass effect caused by an underlying lesion.
- ● In children and adolescents sulci are more difficult to identify, as the parenchymal volume is greater. The superior image slices closer to the vertex are helpful for locating sulci in these age groups.
- ● Uncal herniation is best appreciated in the coronal plane.
- ● Cerebellar tonsillar herniation is best appreciated in the sagittal plane.

Check the parenchymal review areas

At certain sites, subtle pathology may have clinically devastating sequelae:

- ❏ precentral gyrus (motor cortex)
- ❏ postcentral (sensory cortex)
- ❏ basal ganglia
- ❏ internal capsule
- ❏ brain stem
- ❏ pituitary fossa.

Interpretation Tips

Parenchymal review areas

- ● Assessment of the brain stem with CT can be challenging, as it is susceptible to beam-hardening artefact from the adjacent skull base.

Ventricles and other extra-axial CSF spaces

The CSF spaces can be divided into the ventricular system and the other extra-axial CSF spaces.

Is there ventricular enlargement?

An excessive volume of CSF within the cranium is termed 'hydrocephalus'. This can be obstructive (non-communicating) – due to blocked CSF flow – or non-obstructive (communicating) – due to reduced absorption or increased production of CSF. Dilatation of all ventricles implies a non-obstructive cause.

Interpretation Tips

Ventricular enlargement

- ● The temporal horns of the lateral ventricles typically dilate first in early hydrocephalus.
- ● Hydrocephalus may produce transependymal oedema, seen as low attenuation, best appreciated around the temporal, frontal and occipital horns.
- ● Distinguishing between hydrocephalus and prominent ventricles due to generalized parenchymal volume loss in the ageing brain can be difficult. Comparison of the ventricular size with the degree of sulcal widening is key. If ventricular enlargement is disproportionate, hydrocephalus should be suspected.

Is there distortion of the ventricles or other CSF spaces?

The lateral ventricles should be symmetrical. The midline third ventricle should be slit shaped and the fourth ventricle rhomboid shaped on axial images. Any loss of symmetry should be considered abnormal. Any of the ventricles or basal cisterns may be compressed by local mass effect or be dilated by localized hydrocephalus or adjacent volume loss.

Is there blood or debris?

In the patient with headache, fever or impairment of consciousness, look for debris or blood in the subarachnoid space (Fig. 1.6).

Subarachnoid haemorrhage (SAH)

CT has a high sensitivity for detecting SAH within the first 24 hours, decreasing with time. SAH can be subtle, particularly in patients with delayed presentations. Review areas for SAH include:

❑ occipital horns of the lateral ventricles
❑ third ventricle
❑ interpeduncular cistern
❑ prepontine cistern
❑ premedullary cistern
❑ cerebral convexity sulci.

Hydrocephalus may complicate SAH and the ventricular volume must be assessed.

Meningitis

Imaging evidence of meningeal inflammation (with the exception of malignant and tuberculous meningitis) is unusual on CT and MRI. If the CSF contains abnormal cells, these may be seen as intraventricular debris, typically seen lying dependently in the occipital horns (see Fig. 1.6).

Fig. 1.6. The signs of meningitis can be very subtle. The posterior aspect of the occipital horns are usually tapered; however, a flattened appearance is created bilaterally by debris layering dependently within the lateral ventricles (a).

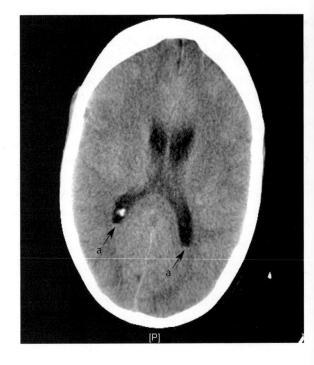

Interpretation Tips

Subarachnoid haemorrhage and intracranial infection

● A subtle focus of high density in the ventricles or basal cisterns may be the only CT evidence of SAH.
● Check the paranasal sinuses, middle-ear clefts and mastoid air cells for potential sources of infection.
● Check for complications of infection, including venous sinus thrombosis and intracranial collections.

Are the ventricles, convexity sulci and basal cisterns poorly visualized?

Ventricular, sulcal and basal cistern effacement raises the possibility of increased intracranial pressure or local mass effect.

The dura, subdural and extradural spaces

Is there haemorrhage?

Check the extra-axial spaces for blood. Distinguishing between subarachnoid, subdural and extradural haemorrhage is important (Table 1.6), as this influences patient management.

Fig. 1.7 demonstrates an example of a subdural haemorrhage.

Table 1.6. Distinguishing between subdural and extradural haemorrhage

Features	Subdural haemorrhage (SDH)	Extradural haemorrhage (EDH)
Clinical	Wide range of presentation: confusion, decreased consciousness, headache, gait disturbance	Typically secondary to head injury, with 80% of cases associated with skull fracture
	Delayed presentation common	A classic latent period may precede rapidly decreasing level of consciousness
CT features	Typical crescent shape over cerebral convexity	Typical biconvex, lentiform shape
	Can cross skull sutures	Restricted by dural tethering at normal cranial sutures
	Bound by meningeal reflections, not crossing the falx and tentorium	Can cross between the skull vault and falx or tentorium
	Will not displace dural venous sinuses away from the skull vault	Can displace dural venous sinuses from the skull vault

Fig. 1.7. Large, isodense subdural haemorrhage on CT (a). The brain is displaced medially (b), causing right lateral ventricular (c) and sulcal effacement. Shallow, isodense collections can be very subtle, so always look for brain parenchyma reaching the inner skull table.

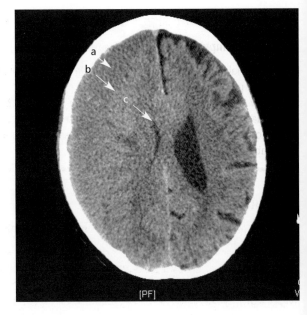

Interpretation Tips

Subdural and extradural haemorrhage

- Shallow subdural haemorrhage can be difficult to identify against the dense skull vault and assessment with wider (e.g. mediastinal) window settings is essential.
- Bilateral subdural haemorrhage can be difficult to diagnose as there is no overall loss of symmetry. This is particularly true of bilateral, isodense subdural haemorrhage, when defining the blood from the convexity cortex is difficult. Look carefully.
- Extradural haemorrhage will not cross normal sutures, but can cross diastased sutures.

Is there evidence of infection?

Check the subdural and extradural spaces for collections.

Subdural empyema
This may be fiendishly subtle, particularly without intravenous contrast. An empyema follows the same rules for the subdural compartment as SDH, but:

- ❏ is typically much smaller and shallower
- ❏ usually has a thin rim of enhancement
- ❏ is often very subtle with CT but is more obvious on MRI.

Extradural abscess
This is usually due to direct spread of infection from the paranasal sinuses, middle-ear clefts or mastoid air cells. If shallow, it may be difficult to distinguish extradural abscess from subdural empyema.

Interpretation Tips

Subdural empyema

● Coronal plane imaging/reformats are helpful for identifying empyema, as a parafalcine position is common.
● Pay particular attention adjacent to the paranasal sinuses, middle-ear clefts and mastoid air cells, which are important sources of infection.
● Look for complications, including venous thrombosis, cerebritis and cerebral abscess.

Vasculature

Is there any evidence of arterial occlusion, dissection or aneurysm?

The unenhanced proximal major intracranial arteries contain flowing blood and are normally slightly denser than brain parenchyma on unenhanced CT. In suspected early stroke, these arteries should be reviewed for evidence of dense thrombus (the 'dense MCA' sign). Basal aneurysms may be seen on unenhanced or post-contrast images.

On conventional MRI sequences, flowing blood within patent arteries should return signal void (i.e. look black). Abnormal signal within the lumen or wall of an artery should raise suspicion.

Is there any evidence of venous sinus thrombosis?

Venous sinus thrombosis (VST) can be a challenging diagnosis to make and the dural venous sinuses and deep venous system are important review areas. As in the major arteries, flowing venous blood is slightly denser than brain parenchyma on unenhanced CT. Increased density within venous structures suggests venous thrombosis. A post-contrast CT or CT venogram may demonstrate thrombus as a filling defect in the vein, or as a complete occlusion of the vessel.

Flowing venous blood returns signal void on conventional MRI sequences. Loss of this signal void suggests venous thrombosis. Dedicated MRI venography sequences may be helpful.

Recognizing features suggestive of VST at presentation is very important. Venous hypertension may lead to infarcts, and then haemorrhage. Suspicious features include:

❏ infarct crossing arterial territories
❏ bilateral infarcts
❏ infarct with acute haemorrhage early in its course
❏ bilateral or multifocal haemorrhage
❏ dense dural venous sinuses or veins on unenhanced CT
❏ expansion of an occluded sinus
❏ loss of normal venous flow void on MRI.

Interpretation Tip

Venous sinus thrombosis

● Normal anatomical variation in the volumes of the right and left transverse and sigmoid sinus systems is a common finding.

Skull, facial bones and mandible

Is there a fracture?

Skull
If a fracture line is identified, it must be followed carefully. Beware of fractures that cross skull base foramina or the middle/inner ear, which raise suspicion of neurovascular injury. Supporting evidence of fractures includes scalp swelling, intracranial air, and blood within the paranasal sinuses, middle-ear cleft or mastoid air cells. Familiarity with the sutures of the skull is essential. Assessment for symmetry is helpful to identify subtle fractures and to prevent sutures being incorrectly identified as fractures.

Interpretation Tips

Skull fracture

● Three-dimensional reformats are useful in identifying fractures of the skull base lying in the axial plane, which are difficult to appreciate on axial imaging.
● Review with a bone algorithm is essential, rather than simply windowing the brain algorithm images.

Facial bones, mandible and temporomandibular joints
The volume of the facial bones and mandible covered varies, but both are important review areas in trauma cases. Look for dislocation of a temporomandibular joint.

Are the paranasal sinuses, middle ear and mastoids normally aerated?

Inflammatory diseases are the commonest cause. Sinusitis, mastoiditis and middle-ear infection are important causes of headache and may also be the source of intracranial infection. Identifying fluid levels may help locate fractures.

Is the bone normal?

Skull metastases are commonly encountered, as well as skull involvement by other bone diseases (e.g. Paget's disease or myeloma – Fig. 1.8).

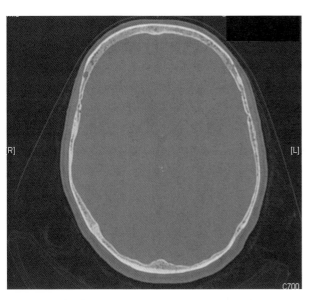

Fig. 1.8. It is important to look at bone algorithms on CT. In this case several small, rounded, lytic lesions within the skull vault revealed an incidental diagnosis of myeloma.

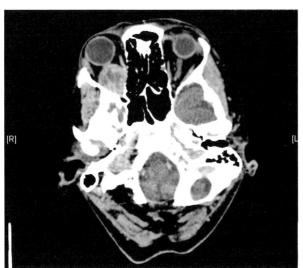

Fig. 1.9. Always review the orbits. This CT scan demonstrates a right retro-orbital secondary breast carcinoma deposit.

Cervical spine

A section of the upper cervical spine is usually included on a CT and MRI brain acquisition. Look for fractures or dislocations.

Orbits

Look for orbital masses (Fig. 1.9), fractures of the orbital margin and evidence of intraorbital infection. Shallow subperiosteal collections may be very subtle and can cause intracranial infection.

Soft tissues

Scalp swelling indicates the location of head trauma and may suggest an underlying injury.

QUICK REFERENCE CHECKLIST

Brain CT and MRI

Images and sequences
Neurosurgical hardware
Brain parenchyma
● Loss of symmetry
● Loss of grey–white differentiation
● Diffuse cerebral swelling
● Focal abnormality – high- or low-density masses
● Mass effect
● Parenchymal review areas
Ventricles and CSF-containing spaces
● Ventricular enlargement
● Ventricular distortion
● Blood or debris
● Poor visualization of CSF spaces
Dural spaces
● Haemorrhage
● Infection
Vasculature
● Arterial occlusion, dissection or aneurysm
● Venous sinus thrombosis
Skull, facial bones and mandible
● Fractures, sinuses and bone quality
Cervical spine
Orbits
Soft tissues

HEAD AND NECK RADIOLOGY (2)

FACIAL RADIOGRAPHS

Mid-facial injuries are best assessed with the occipito-mental (OM) and occipito-mental 30° (OM30) views. Facial views can be difficult to interpret because of the presence of overlapping bones, soft tissues and air.

Soft-tissue swelling

Look for unilateral soft-tissue swelling, indicating the site of potential bone injury.

McGrigor's lines

Follow these three lines looking for fractures (Fig. 2.1). Compare both sides of the face when looking for subtle fractures.

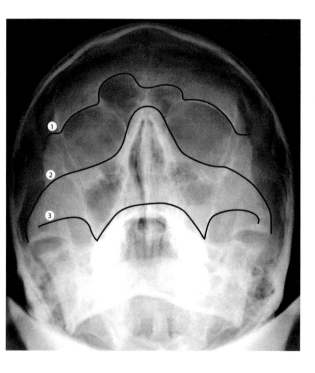

Fig. 2.1. McGrigor's lines. Note the fluid level within the left maxillary antrum: in the context of trauma, this raises the possibility of occult fracture.

❏ *Line 1*. Start at the zygomaticofrontal suture, looking for widening. Follow along the supraorbital margins and note whether there is any fluid in the frontal sinus.
❏ *Line 2*. Start at the superior border of the zygomatic arch and follow across the zygoma and infraorbital margin, and over the contour of the nasal bone.
❏ *Line 3*. Follow the inferior border of the zygomatic arch, down the lateral border of the maxillary antrum, along the inferior margin of the antrum and the roots of the teeth within the maxilla.

If one fracture is identified, continue to search for additional fractures (Fig. 2.2).

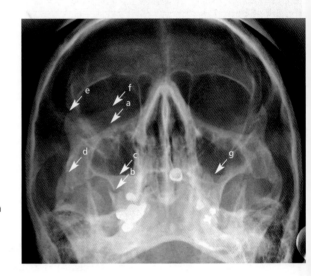

Fig. 2.2. A fracture at one site should prompt the search for another. Here there is a right orbital floor fracture (a), fracture of the lateral wall of the right maxillary antrum (b), with an associated fluid level (c), fracture of the right zygomatic arch (d), and diastasis of the right zygamaticofrontal suture (e). Also note the soft-tissue swelling projected over the right eye (f) and the fluid level within the left maxillary antrum (g).

Maxillary sinuses

Here look for:

❏ a fluid level within the sinus, which indicates haemorrhage following fracture (although fluid levels can be seen in non-traumatic conditions such as sinusitis)
❏ mucosal thickening and polyps
❏ the 'teardrop' sign of herniation of orbital contents into the maxillary sinus following an orbital floor blow-out fracture (Fig. 2.3).

Orbits

If the preceding search has failed to reveal any orbital injury, look for the black 'eyebrow' sign of free intraorbital air following fracture.

Foreign bodies

If indicated by the history, check for radio-opaque densities within the orbits and soft tissues.

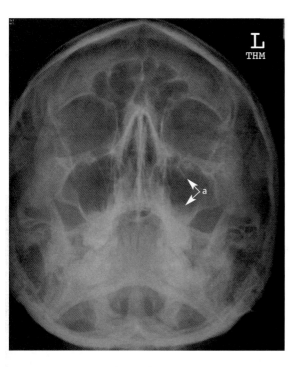

Fig. 2.3. Teardrop fracture of the left orbital floor: herniation of orbital contents into the left maxillary antrum with an associated fluid level (a).

Interpretation Tips

Facial radiograph

● It may be difficult to see McGrigors's lines 2 and 3 if the head is not tilted correctly, or difficult to trace on one side if the image is rotated.
● Isolated fractures of the zygomatic arch are common, but, if a more complex injury is suspected, have a low threshold for CT.

QUICK REFERENCE CHECKLIST

Facial radiograph

Soft-tissue swelling
McGrigor's lines
Maxillary sinuses
Orbits
Foreign bodies

ORTHOPANTOMOGRAM (OPG)

The mandible acts as a bony ring, so, if one fracture is seen, suspect a second injury (Fig. 2.4).

Fig. 2.4. The right-sided mandibular fracture is easy to see. Have a low index of suspicion for a second fracture, in this case through the left mandibular ramus.

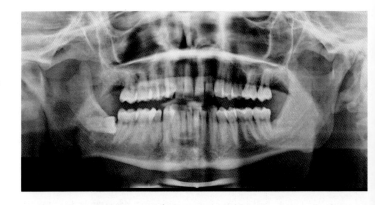

Mandibular contour

Follow the lower mandibular border, then trace the outline of the condyles and coronoid processes, looking for fractures.

Temporomandibular joints

Check for dislocation of the temporomandibular joints.

Teeth

Look for fractured or missing teeth as well as lucent lesions (e.g. abscesses around the dental roots).

Dental occlusion

The spacing between the upper and lower teeth should be equal; if it is not, this suggests a condylar neck fracture with shortening.

Interpretation Tips

Orthopantomogram

● As air from the orophaynx is projected over the angle of the mandible, beware of over-calling fractures by checking the contralateral side for comparison, and checking that disruption does not extend beyond the bone margin.

● Although the orthopantomogram is ideally suited to identifying dental abnormalities and abnormalities of the temporomandibular joints, it is often requested for fractures; however, as it is a tomogram, undisplaced fractures may be 'blurred' out. If a fracture is suspected, but not clearly identified, recommend further oblique and PA views of the mandible.

THYROID AND NECK ULTRASOUND

The commonest indication for thyroid ultrasound is to confirm the presence of a goitre and establish its cause. If malignancy is suspected fine-needle aspiration or core biopsy will need to be performed. As well as the gland, complete examination should also encompass other anterior neck structures, as outlined in this suggested review system.

First, assess the thyroid in transverse section with a high-frequency linear probe. Scan from the base of the neck to the submental area. If the whole gland cannot be viewed by midline scanning, scan each lobe in turn. Next, scan each lobe in longitudinal section. Once the thyroid has been examined, scan in transverse section from the base of the neck up to the submandibular glands on each side. If any abnormalities are identified, investigate them further with supplemental longitudinal views. A normal transverse view of the thyroid gland and related structures is demonstrated in Fig. 2.5.

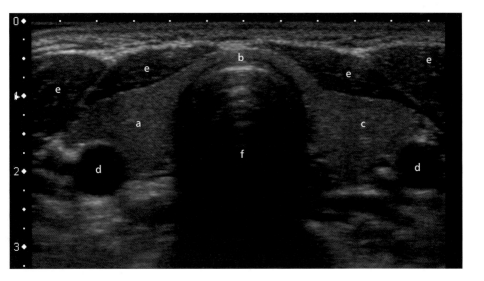

Fig. 2.5. Normal transverse view of the thyroid demonstrating homogeneous high reflectivity relative to surrounding muscle. Right lobe (a), isthmus (b), left lobe (c), carotid arteries (d), strap muscles of the neck (e) and trachea (f).

Thyroid gland

Size

Comment on the size of the gland and the presence of any retrosternal extension or presence of a pyramidal lobe. Diffuse increase in size can indicate thyroiditis. Conversely, a small gland may indicate previous surgery or burnt-out thyroiditis.

Reflectivity

Comment on the overall glandular reflectivity. The thyroid normally displays a homogeneous increased reflectivity compared with surrounding neck structures. Globally reduced reflectivity can indicate thyroiditis.

Vascularity

Assess overall vascularity: decide whether it is normal, increased (e.g. acute thyroiditis) or decreased (rare, e.g. burnt-out Hashimoto's thyroiditis).

Focal nodules

Describe the number and size of nodules. Most thyroid cancers are solitary (one in five solitary nodules is malignant), but a malignant nodule in a multinodular goitre is well recognized. No one feature is diagnostic of cancer. Assess the following to help decide whether a lesion warrants biopsy:

❏ *Reflectivity*. Most, but not all, malignant nodules display overall low heterogeneous reflectivity.
❏ *Presence of cystic elements*. The presence of cystic elements generally indicates a benign aetiology, but up to a third of papillary cancers display cystic areas.
❏ *Calcification*. Malignant calcification tends to be fine throughout the lesion (microcalcifications), whereas benign calcification tends to be coarser and more peripheral.
❏ *Comet tail sign*. This refers to artefact produced distal to high-reflectivity foci in benign colloid nodules which resembles a comet's tail (not to be confused with calcification).
❏ *Halo*. Look for a peripheral halo of lower reflectivity around a nodule representing a capsule. This is generally, but not exclusively, an indication of a benign aetiology.
❏ *Vascularity*. Use Doppler to identify intranodular flow, which indicates malignancy. Benign lesions tend to be avascular or display a peripheral pattern of blood flow.
❏ *Associated lymph nodes*. Check for abnormal lymph nodes; nodal metastases from thyroid cancer are common.

Figs 2.6 and 2.7 demonstrate examples of benign and malignant focal nodules, respectively.

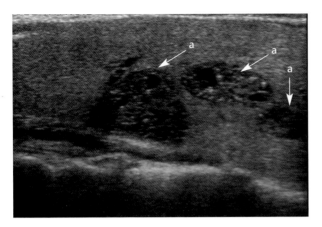

Fig. 2.6. Longitudinal view of the right lobe of the thyroid, demonstrating three well-defined typical colloid nodules (a), containing cystic spaces and thick septa.

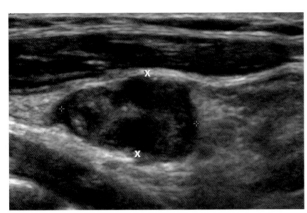

Fig. 2.7. Solitary, low-reflectivity lesion within the thyroid, demonstrating ill-defined internal architecture. Fine-needle aspiration confirmed papillary thyroid carcinoma.

Parathyroid glands

Although normal parathyroid glands are not well seen on ultrasound, the presence of any low-reflectivity lesion posterior to the inferior or superior poles of the thyroid should raise suspicion of parathyroid adenoma.

Vocal cords

The vocal cords are seen in transverse section. Check that they are symmetrical and that both move on phonation. Absence of symmetrical movement indicates vocal cord palsy.

Neck vessels

It is beyond the scope of this section to cover carotid artery and jugular vein pathology in detail, but scan up the anterolateral neck and note any gross carotid stenotic lesions due to atherosclerotic disease. Also note whether there is any echogenic material within the internal jugular vein, as this will indicate established thrombus.

Lymph nodes

No one criterion can reliably differentiate benign from malignant lymphadenopathy. Table 2.1 summarizes the typical features of benign and malignant nodes to guide the decision whether to biopsy.

Table 2.1. The typical features of benign and malignant lymph nodes

	Echotexture	Size	Shape	Echo-genic hilum	Capsular breach	Calcifi-cation	Vascularity
Benign	Homogeneous	Generally smaller	Oval, elongated	Present	Capsule intact	Absent	Organized, hilar
Malignant	Heterogeneous	Generally larger	Rounded	Absent	Capsule breached	Punctuate calcification (metastatic thyroid papillary cancer)	Disorganized, peripheral

Figs 2.8 and 2.9 demonstrate examples of typical benign and malignant lymph nodes, respectively.

Submandibular glands

Finally, evaluate the submandibular glands. Note low-reflectivity intraglandular lesions. If there is distal dilatation, search for a cause such as an echogenic calculus. If the gland is small, atrophic and avascular, consider inflammatory conditions such as sarcoidosis and Sjögren's syndrome.

Fig. 2.8. Normal, oval lymph nodes, displaying (a) a smooth capsular margin and (b) fatty hila.

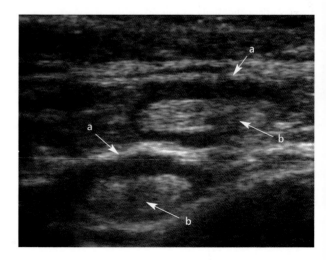

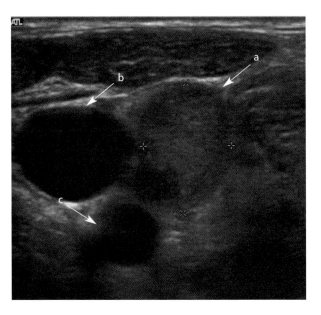

Fig. 2.9. Abnormal rounded and enlarged neck lymph node displaying mixed internal reflectivity (a) adjacent to the internal jugular vein (b) and carotid artery (c), in this case secondary to thyroid carcinoma.

Interpretation Tips

Thyroid and neck ultrasound

● Place a pillow under the patient's shoulders to extend the neck during scanning.
● Remember, no single ultrasound feature is diagnostic of malignancy; rather, use the constellation of findings to guide a decision whether to biopsy or not.
● It is often difficult to visualize the vocal cords in older male patients owing to the presence of thyroid cartilage and tracheal ring calcification.

QUICK REFERENCE CHECKLIST

Thyroid and neck ultrasound

Thyroid
● Size
● Reflectivity
● Vascularity
● Nodules
  – Reflectivity
  – Cystic elements
  – Calcification
  – Comet tail sign
  – Halo
  – Vascularity
  – Associated lymph nodes

continued

QUICK REFERENCE CHECKLIST *continued*

Parathyroid glands
Vocal cords
Neck vessels
Lymph nodes
● Echotexture
● Size
● Shape
● Echogenic hilum
● Capsular breach
● Calcification
● Vascularity
Submandibular glands

IMAGING OF THE EXTRACRANIAL HEAD AND NECK

Understanding the complex anatomy in this area can greatly aid image interpretation. Diagnosis of head and neck disorders involves input from clinicians, radiologists and pathologists. The diagnosis has often been made by clinicians, and imaging is used as a problem solver, to identify a clinically occult lesion and to define disease extent.

As well as imaging features, a number of non-imaging factors can narrow the differential diagnosis, and these are included in the review system set out here.

The patient with a lump in the neck

Age

The majority of neck masses in children are congenital or developmental, whereas there is an increased incidence of inflammatory or neoplastic masses in adults.

Site

The location of a mass can significantly narrow the differential diagnosis. Layers of deep cervical fascia divide the neck into a number of spaces. Pathology is confined to the limited number of structures that occupy each space (Table 2.2). These facial spaces of the neck are shown in Fig. 2.10.

The parapharyngeal space, deep in the neck, is related on all sides to four other spaces of the neck. Masses arising from surrounding spaces leave characteristic impressions upon the parapharyngeal space, facilitating identification of the space of origin of a mass. Table 2.3 lists the imaging features of masses originating in the different fascial spaces of the neck.

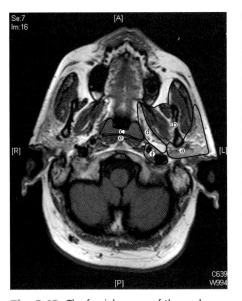

Fig. 2.10. The fascial spaces of the neck. Parotid space (a), masticator space (b), mucosal space (c), parapharyngeal space (d), retropharyngeal space (e) and carotid space (f).

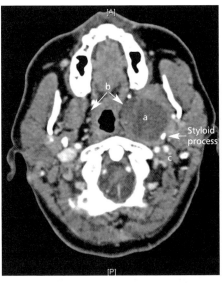

Fig. 2.11. Evaluation of the site of origin of a mass. Note the large mass (a) in the deep tissues of the neck. Note how the mass compresses the parapharyngeal fat (b) on its lateral surface and displaces it medially. Also note how the vessels of the carotid sheath (c) are displaced slightly posteriorly. This is consistent with a mass arising in the parotid space, in this case a parotid carcinoma. Styloid process is arrowed.

Table 2.2. The spaces comprising the layers of deep cervical fascia

Space	Description
Mucosal	Mucosa of the upper aerodigestive tract
Carotid	Extends from skull base to aortic arch and contains structures of the carotid sheath
Parotid	Contains the parotid gland and lymph nodes
Masticator	Extends from the angle of the mandible to the temporalis muscle, and contains the muscles of mastication
Parapharyngeal	Runs vertically from the skull base to the hyoid bone. The tough pharyngobasilar fascia forms its medial border, separating it from the mucosal space. Once this layer is breached, the parapharyngeal space serves as an important conduit for infection in the neck
Retropharyngeal	A posterior potential midline space lying posterior to the mucosal space and anterior to the prevertebral space. Extends inferiorly to the superior mediastinum, and so serves as an important conduit for infection

Table 2.3. The imaging features of masses originating in the different fascial spaces of the neck

Space	Constituents	Mass effect on the parapharyngeal space	Comments
Mucosal	Mucosa, lymphoid tissue, salivary glands	Displaces laterally	
Carotid	Vessels, carotid body, cranial nerves IX–XII, sympathetic chain, lymph nodes	Displaces anteriorly	Masses may displace the styloid process anteriorly
Parotid	Parotid gland, lymph nodes, vessels, facial nerve	Displaces medially	Masses push the styloid process and carotid vessels posteriorly
Masticator	Muscle, bone, branches of cranial nerve V3	Displaces posteromedially	Site of tumour extension. Beware of perineural extension (nerve V3) to skull base
Parapharyngeal	Fat, cranial nerve V3, vessels		Route of infection spread
Retropharyngeal	Fat, lymph nodes		Common site of nodal metastases. Route of infection to the mediastinum

The parapharyngeal space serves as an important indicator of mass effect in the neck. Fig. 2.11 demonstrates the effect of a mass on the parapharyngeal space.

Solid or cystic

Ultrasound is useful for characterizing the nature of masses.

> *Interpretation Tips*
>
> **Solid or cystic masses**
>
> ● A laterally placed cystic mass in a young adult is most commonly a branchial cyst.
> ● Masses in the midline, especially in children or young adults, are usually either developmental or related to the thyroid.
> ● A laterally placed solid mass in an adult is usually an enlarged lymph node and should prompt the search for an inflammatory or neoplastic cause.

Results of a fine-needle aspirate (FNA)

Adult patients with enlarged lymph nodes will commonly undergo an FNA. Cervical lymphadenopathy can be reactive, neoplastic or secondary to connective-tissue disorder. Most of these patients will have a primary malignancy discovered on a focused ENT clinical examination. There is, however, a subset of patients whose diagnosis will be suggested by imaging.

Interpretation Tips

Carcinoma in the neck

● Sometimes imaging of the neck fails to reveal a primary cancer. Positron emission tomography (PET), sometimes combined with a CT scan, can increase the chance of detection.

● Lung and skin carcinoma (melanoma or SCC) commonly give rise to metastatic adenopathy in the neck.

Lymph node FNA reveals squamous cell carcinoma (SCC)

The most common sites for SCC in the extracranial head and neck are the base of tongue, the nasopharynx, the tonsil and larynx.

Tongue base

Unfortunately, the tongue base is difficult to image on CT, as much of it is often obscured secondary to beam-hardening artefact from dental amalgam. MRI is therefore useful in assessing this area.

Nasopharynx

The most common histological subtype of carcinoma in the nasopharynx in the UK is SCC. Assess two key sites for a mass lesion, effacement or asymmetry:

❏ the lateral pharyngeal recess (fossa of Rosenmüller)
❏ the opening of the pharyngotympanic (eustachian) tube.

The fossa of Rosenmüller is difficult to visualize adequately on nasendoscopy. Fig. 2.12 demonstrates asymmetry of the fossa of Rosenmüller.

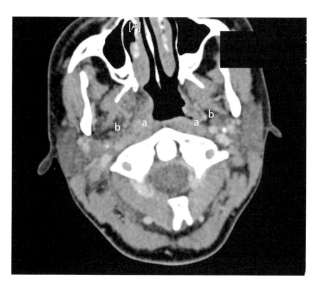

Fig. 2.12. Asymmetry of the fossa of Rosenmüller. Note effacement of the right lateral pharyngeal recess (a). Note that the right-sided parapharyngeal fat (b) is of greater density than that on the other side, in this case owing to an invasive nasopharyngeal carcinoma. (Both sides marked for comparison.)

Interpretation Tips

Scans of the nasopharynx

● The eustachian tube can be obstructed by a nasopharyngeal tumour, leading to accumulation of fluid in the middle ear.

● Although it can be a normal feature, asymmetry of the lateral pharyngeal recess should prompt a targeted examination.

● The presence of a thin line of mucosal enhancement on contrast-enhanced T1-weighted MR scans in an effaced lateral pharyngeal recess is suggestive of benign adenoidal enlargement.

● The pterygopalatine fossa usually contains a variable amount of fat. Soft tissue here implies tumour involvement. The ptergyopalatine fossa has communications with the orbit and middle cranial fossa; thus, tumour involvement here implies non-resectable disease.

Tonsil

Tonsillar tumours can be difficult to recognize on imaging owing to:

❏ normal asymmetry
❏ infective disease of the tonsil mimicking malignancy
❏ poor enhancement of small tumours.

Larynx

Carcinomas of the larynx are usually detected on endoscopic examination. The key aspects to assess are:

❏ involvement of the paraglottic spaces (SCC here can spread via the submucosal route in a cranial or caudal direction)
❏ the presence of laryngeal cartilage invasion
❏ involvement of the anterior commissure (in SCC of the vocal cords, thickening of the anterior commissure implies disease involvement across the midline, which has important prognostic implications).

Interpretation Tip

Scans of the larynx

● The variable nature of laryngeal cartilage ossification and inflammatory changes in the larynx may make subtle invasion of the laryngeal cartilage difficult to identify radiologically.

Lymph node FNA reveals lymphoma

Histologically, lymphoma can be classified as either Hodgkin's lymphoma or non-Hodgkin's lymphoma. Lymphoma can be either nodal or extranodal. Extranodal lymphoma is more common in non-Hodgkin's lymphoma.

The radiological differentiation of lymphoma and SCC can be difficult. Lymphoma is suggested by:

❏ non-necrotic lymph node involvement
❏ a multicentric distribution of disease
❏ less propensity for bone destruction
❏ multiple, bilateral, non-contiguous sites of lymph node involvement
❏ involvement of Waldeyer's lymphatic ring, often with extension into the nasopharynx, which can lead to airway obstruction
❏ lymph node enlargement in the thorax and abdomen, with splenomegaly.

QUICK REFERENCE CHECKLIST

The patient with a lump in the neck

Patient age
Site
● fascial space of origin
Solid or cystic (ultrasound)
FNA results to guide image interpretation
● SCC
  – Tongue base
  – Nasopharynx
  – Tonsil
  – Larynx
● Lymphoma

THE IMAGING OF HEARING LOSS

Hearing loss can be conductive, sensorineural or mixed. As always, familiarity with anatomy is important. Comparison with the contralateral side is helpful.

Conductive hearing loss

This is usually due to disease of the external ear, tympanic membrane or ossicular chain. CT is the preferred method of investigation. Cholesteatoma is arguably the most important disease in this group and recognition is vital to enable early initiation of treatment. The diagnosis is suggested by a combination of history, audiometry and otoscopic examination. Aim to answer the following questions.

Is there a cholesteatoma?

Cholesteatoma is soft-tissue density on CT, and is often difficult to differentiate from granulation tissue or debris. Cholesteatoma is suggested by:

❑ evidence of bone erosion
❑ poor pneumatization of the mastoid
❑ non-dependent homogeneous mass
❑ no enhancement (granulation tissue may enhance).

Cholesteatoma most commonly originates from Prussak's space (between the pars flaccida of the tympanic membrane and the neck of the malleus).

An example of cholesteatoma is demonstrated in Fig. 2.13.

If there is a cholesteatoma, what is the disease extent?

Look for bone erosion suggested by focal demineralization. Important bones include:

❑ scutum (an early sign of cholesteatoma)
❑ ossicular chain
❑ bony labyrinth (involvement of the bone prominence caused by the lateral semi-circular canal in the medial wall of the middle ear is an early sign of labyrinthine involvement).

Also check the prominence of the facial nerve canal in the middle ear and assess the tegmen tympani, the roof of the middle ear, which can provide a path for spread of infection into the middle cranial fossa.

Is there evidence of otospongiosis or sclerosis?

This is an important cause of hearing loss and usually presents with either conductive or mixed hearing loss, which is commonly bilateral. The diagnosis is often missed on CT as the findings can be subtle. The earliest radiological finding is of spongiotic new bone transformation, which manifests radiologically as demineralization of the normally dense petrous bone.

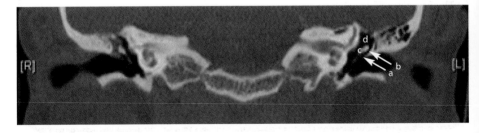

Fig. 2.13. Right cholesteatoma. Note confluent soft tissue that widens Prussak's space and fills the attic. There is truncation of the scutum and displacement of the ossicular chain. The contralateral side is labelled for reference: scutum (a), Prussak's space (b), ossicular chain (c), attic (d).

Sensorineural hearing loss

This is usually due to disease of the inner ear or the vestibulocochlear nerve and pathways. Many microscopic abnormalities are not visible on imaging, although an identifiable cause may be apparent, such as a vestibular schwannoma.

Vestibular schwannoma

Some 95% of schwannomas are unilateral. Bilateral schwannomas are diagnostic of type 2 neurofibromatosis. MRI is the investigation of choice. Look for:

❏ low-signal, well-circumscribed, CSF-filling defect along the path of nerve VIII on T2-weighted images (small tumours)
❏ avid enhancement on CT or gadolinium-enhanced, T1-weighted sequences.

Secondary effects from larger tumours include:

❏ enlargement of internal auditory canal
❏ cerebellopontine angle cistern effacement
❏ effacement of the fourth ventricle, with or without hydrocephalus.

Post-meningitic hearing loss

Post-meningitic hearing loss can be a result of ossification of the structures of the inner ear, termed 'labyrinthitis ossificans'. This may be suggested by:

❏ ossification of the inner ear on CT (late disease)
❏ loss of labyrinth fluid signal on T2-weighted MR images (early disease).

Post-traumatic hearing loss

This is usually due to an injury to the inner ear or vestibulocochlear nerve as a result of a fracture of the temporal bone.

QUICK REFERENCE CHECKLIST

The imaging of hearing loss

Conductive loss
● Cholesteatoma
Sensorineural hearing loss
● Vestibular schwannoma
● Post-meningitic hearing loss
● Post-traumatic hearing loss

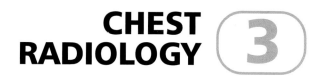
FRONTAL CHEST RADIOGRAPH

The frontal chest radiograph is one of the most frequently requested investigations, and yet it is one of the most difficult to interpret.

Technical factors

❏ *Projection*. Check whether the film has been taken anteroposteriorly (image plate behind patient) or posteroanteriorly (image plate in front of patient). On the PA projection, the scapulae are generally positioned laterally and do not overlie the lungs. AP projections can artificially magnify structures towards the front of the chest, such as the heart. Also check whether the film was taken with the patient erect or supine.

❏ *Rotation*. Ensure that the medial ends of the clavicles are equidistant from the spinous processes.

❏ *Orientation*. Check the markings for left and right.

❏ *Penetration*. Is the image over-penetrated (too dark), under-penetrated (too white) or adequate (vertebral bodies just visible behind the heart)?

❏ *Inspiration*. The anterior end of the sixth rib, or the posterior end of the tenth, should be above the diaphragm. If less is visible of either rib, this equates to a poor inspiration; if more is visible, this points to hyperinflation.

Trachea

The trachea normally passes slightly to the right of the midline. Tracheal position can be altered; for instance it will be pulled over by reduced lung volume, and pushed over by a superior mediastinal mass. The carinal angle should be approximately 60–75°, but can be widened in subcarinal lymphadenopathy or left atrial enlargement.

Heart and mediastinum

Review the cardiac outline and evaluate the size of the heart, which should not exceed half the trans-thoracic diameter. Beware apparent false enlargement with poor inspiration, AP projection or supine positioning.

Look at the right heart border, made up of the right atrium. Above the right hilum the superior vena cava forms the right mediastinal border.

Fig. 3.1. Rounded lung metastases secondary to oesophageal adenocarcinoma. The distal oesophageal stent seen behind the heart strongly suggests an oesophageal primary tumour.

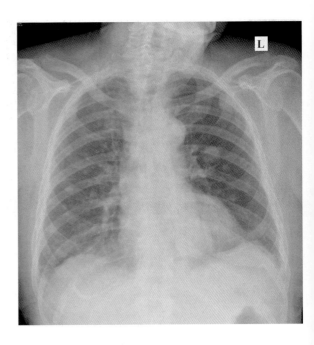

The left heart border represents the left ventricular outline. If the normal concavity is lost between the hilum and the left ventricular border, this indicates enlargement of the left atrial appendage. Above the left hilum, formed by the left pulmonary artery, evaluate the size and shape of the aortic knuckle.

Finally, look carefully for densities projected behind the cardiac silhouette (Fig. 3.1).

Hila

The left hilum lies up to 2 cm above the right hilum. Assess hilar shape, size and density.

Lungs

Look for discrete or diffuse opacity. Try to determine whether opacification represents alveolar or interstitial shadowing. It is helpful to compare both lungs, zone by zone, not neglecting the apices. Assess vascular markings and bronchi, and look for either focal or global volume loss. Beware that problems in the breasts, soft tissues and ribs can masquerade as lung pathology. Identify the horizontal fissure, which on the PA view runs from the right hilum to the region of the sixth rib in the axillary line.

Pleura

Look for a subtle pneumothorax. Record the presence of an effusion, even if small. Identify pleural thickening or plaque, which may or may not be calcified. Classic

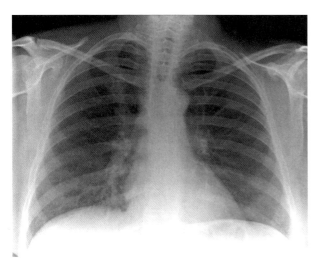

Fig. 3.2. On first glance, this chest radiograph looks normal; however, systematic review reveals erosion of the anterior left second rib, with a subtle associated soft-tissue mass.

calcified plaques due to asbestos exposure are often described as 'holly leaf' in shape due to their sharply defined, angular borders.

Diaphragms and costophrenic angles

The right hemidiaphragm usually lies above the left. Loss of definition suggests lower lobe collapse or consolidation. Look for free gas beneath the diaphragm. Look for abnormal bowel gas patterns.

Bones

Review all the bones, paying particular attention to the ribs, for fractures or destructive lesions (Fig. 3.2).

Soft tissues

Check soft tissues for swelling or subcutaneous emphysema. Ensure that both breasts are visible on female patients.

Review areas

Finally, re-examine the areas where pathology is commonly missed:

- ❏ lung apices
- ❏ behind the heart
- ❏ hila
- ❏ behind and below the hemidiaphragms
- ❏ bones.

Methodical review of the image may reveal a unifying diagnosis (Fig. 3.3).

Fig. 3.3. Perihilar interstitial thickening and Kerley B lines (a). The previous right mastectomy and right axillary lymph node dissection clips point to the diagnosis: lymphangitis carcinomatosis secondary to breast carcinoma. There is also an incidental fracture of the right clavicle.

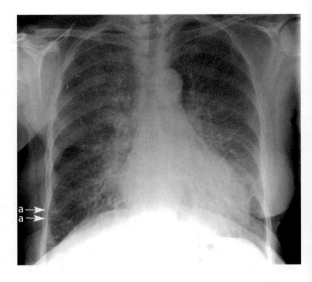

Interpretation Tips

Frontal chest radiograph

- Air bronchograms indicate that shadowing is intrapulmonary.
- Areas where common pathology is often missed include: lung apices, behind the heart, hila, behind and below the hemidiaphragms, bones.

QUICK REFERENCE CHECKLIST

Frontal chest radiograph

Technical factors
Trachea
Heart and mediastinum
Hila
Lungs
Pleura
Diaphragms and costophrenic angles
Bones
Soft tissues
Review areas

LATERAL CHEST RADIOGRAPH

The lateral chest radiograph is rarely interpreted in isolation, but does prove a useful adjunct to the frontal radiograph in some situations, such as when the exact location of a lung parenchymal lesion is to be determined.

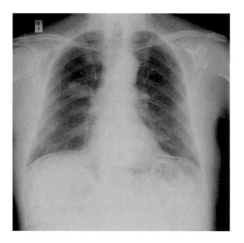

Fig. 3.4. A frontal radiograph (patient erect) reveals pneumoperitoneum in addition to an incidental right-sided lung cancer.

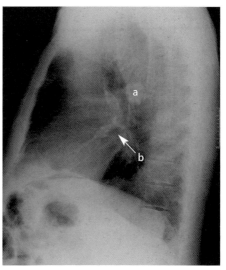

Fig. 3.5. The lateral image from the same patient as in Fig. 3.4 demonstrates the lesion (a) above the oblique fissure (b) within the right upper lobe.

Identify the right and left hemidiaphragms

The left hemidiaphragm can be distinguished from the right as the heart will obliterate its anterior portion, and a gastric air bubble may be identified beneath it. The inferior vena cava (IVC) may be seen to pierce the right hemidiaphragm. Once identified, check for free sub-diaphragmatic air.

Lungs

Look in front, above and behind the cardiac shadow, paying particular attention to the retrosternal air space for anteriorly placed lesions. Also actively look for pathology behind the diaphragms and in the costophrenic angles.

Fissures

Identify the horizontal fissure. The oblique fissures arise at the T4–5 vertebrae and pass inferiorly to the hemidiaphragm. Once these landmarks have been identified, localizing a lesion seen initially on the frontal radiograph is relatively straightforward (Figs 3.4 and 3.5).

Hila

Check the size and density of the hila, ensuring that there is no central mass lesion.

Pleura

Look for effusions and pleural thickening. Calcified plaques, often most florid on the hemidiaphragms, indicate previous asbestos exposure.

Heart

An enlarged right ventricle can obliterate the space behind the sternum. Left atrial enlargement gives a rounded appearance of the posterior cardiac silhouette. Valvular calcification can be seen on the lateral radiograph and should be recorded.

Vertebrae

Check the height and alignment of the vertebral bodies. Normally the lower thoracic vertebrae appear more translucent than the upper vertebrae. If they appear denser, suspect consolidation or atelectasis within the lower lobes.

QUICK REFERENCE CHECKLIST

Lateral chest radiograph

Identify the right and left diaphragms
Lungs
Fissures
Hila
Pleura
Heart
Vertebrae

CHEST CT

First look at the lungs and airways on dedicated lung windows, changing to mediastinal windows to look at the remainder of the chest. Finally, change to bone windows to assess the skeleton.

Technical parameters

Note the following:

❏ whether the image is contrast enhanced
❏ the phase of image acquisition post-contrast (i.e. pulmonary arterial, arterial or delayed)
❏ whether the neck, abdomen or pelvis is included.

Technical limitations

Comment on the adequacy of contrast, or whether there is significant motion artefact from breathing.

Lung windows

Lungs

Altered attenuation

Note any difference in the pattern of attenuation between the lungs. Note whether or not this conforms to lung segmental anatomy. If there is a difference in transradiancy between hemithoraces, then look carefully for signs of volume loss. Clues include splaying of the vascular structures and displacement of the interlobar fissures on the affected side. An atelectatic lobe may be discernible only as a thin opacity when the volume loss is complete, so look carefully.

If there is a patchy pattern of difference in attenuation (mosaic attenuation), try to work out if this is due to:

❏ perfusional abnormality, that is, reduced blood flow (e.g. pulmonary embolism)
❏ airways disease, that is, trapped air – expiratory high-resolution scanning may help demonstrate an increase in differential attenuation between affected and non-affected areas of lung (i.e. apparently blacker areas of lung whereby air is trapped on expiration due to small airway disease)
❏ filling of the airspaces by fluid, debris or cells.

Consolidation

Comment on consolidation as suggested by parenchymal opacification with little volume loss and the presence of air bronchograms. Airspace opacification with underlying lung architecture and vessels still visible within it is termed 'ground-glass' change.

Emphysema

Comment on the presence of emphysema and its distribution, extent and severity.

Nodules and masses

Divide the lung into zones and look for parenchymal nodules (2–30 mm diameter) and masses (≥30 mm diameter).

If there are nodules or masses, note the following:

❏ their number
❏ their attenuation characteristics (e.g. calcification, fat, soft tissue, gas, fluid)
❏ their distribution (i.e. central, peripheral or subpleural)
❏ their morphology (smooth, irregular or spiculated)
❏ any enhancement following contrast
❏ any distortion of the surrounding parenchymal architecture
❏ any effect on, or adherence to, adjacent structures.

Interstitium

Look for septal line thickening and note the following:

❏ whether the thickening is smooth, irregular or beaded (this indicates whether it is due to fluid, fibrosis or infiltration)

❏ its distribution (i.e. basal, upper zone, subpleural or central)
❏ any accompanying 'ground-glass' change.

The identification of these features may point towards a specific diagnosis.

Airways

Note the size and position of the trachea. Follow the individual airways out to the periphery and note any obvious airway luminal narrowing caused by extrinsic compression, wall thickening or intraluminal obstruction by inspissated mucus or soft-tissue mass.

The airways normally taper towards the periphery. Bronchiectasis is diagnosed if the airway is larger in internal diameter than the corresponding vessel.

Small, branching, ill-defined densities ('tree in bud' appearance) in a subpleural location represent centrilobular airways filled with debris and are often indicative of infection, for example tuberculosis.

Mediastinal windows

Pleura

Evaluate the pleura for nodules, plaques, calcification and thickening. The pleura should normally be pencil thin, so compare both sides. Thickening of the mediastinal pleura is especially significant and can indicate mesothelioma. Note air or fluid within the pleural space (pneumothorax and effusion, respectively). Check whether the fluid is of water density or higher (e.g. pus or blood).

Mediastinum and hila

Carefully scrutinize the mediastinum and hila for masses and lymphadenopathy. Lymph nodes are generally measured in their short axis and should be <1 cm (subcarinal nodes <1.5 cm). Assess the effect of any mass on adjacent structures, particularly the airways and the pulmonary vessels. Assess the oesophagus and note any abnormal dilatation or wall thickening.

Heart and vessels

Precise assessment of thoracic vascular anatomy is usually achieved by threshold-triggered scanning (e.g. in pulmonary angiography and aortography). The heart is best examined by ECG-gated cardiac imaging.

Aorta

Begin by assessing the calibre of the aorta. Comment on aneurysmal enlargement, calcification or thrombus. Aberrant vessels arising from the aortic arch are common.

Pulmonary arteries

Next, follow the pulmonary arterial vasculature methodically to the periphery and note any evidence of thromboembolic disease. If embolus is present, comment on:

❑ the site (central, peripheral, bilateral)
❑ whether it is occlusive or non-occlusive
❑ signs of right heart strain – bowing or flattening of the interventricular septum towards the left, or the presence of contrast within the IVC (which suggests tricuspid regurgitation).

Heart and coronary arteries

Note the presence of any coronary artery calcification. Valvular calcification should also be recorded. Assess the pericardium for evidence of pericardial thickening (≥3 mm) and effusion. Look for dilatation of the cardiac chambers and evidence of focal myocardial thinning, which would indicate previous infarction.

Soft tissues

Most imaging protocols will include a variable amount of the neck. Assess the thyroid gland for mass lesions. Pay particular attention to the supraclavicular and axillary lymph node groups, as these may be sites of nodal metastases and lymphoma. Occasionally, an incidental breast mass may be detected (Fig. 3.6).

Below the diaphragm

Most protocols include a variable amount of the abdomen and it is vital to look for abdominal pathology. This is covered in Chapter 5 (see pp. 70–84).

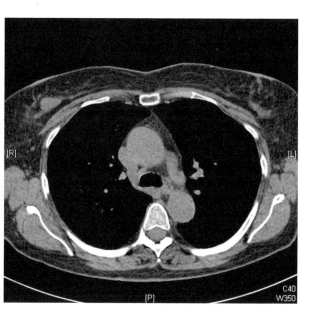

Fig. 3.6. Remember to look at the soft tissues. In this case an incidental right breast lesion is apparent.

Bone windows

Bones

Assess the skeleton for fractures and lesions. While careful appraisal of the bones can be tedious, no one else will check this area and occasionally an unexpected diagnosis can be made.

Interpretation Tips

Chest CT

- Look for isolated parenchymal nodules.
- Tease out the cause of mosaic attenuation.
- Check the soft tissues – supraclavicular area, axillae and breasts.
- Look for thyroid and supraclavicular pathology.
- Do not miss pulmonary emboli when the diagnosis is not suspected (Figs 3.7 and 3.8).

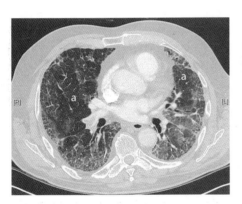 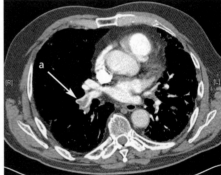

Fig. 3.7. CT to assess worsening breathlessness. The lung window revealed coarsened septal thickening and traction bronchiectasis and bronchiolectasis in a predominantly subpleural distribution. The lower-attenuation areas represent air trapping (a).

Fig. 3.8. CT to assess worsening breathlessness. Changing to mediastinal windows demonstrated an unexpected pulmonary embolus (a).

QUICK REFERENCE CHECKLIST

Chest CT

Technical parameters
Technical limitations
Lung windows
● Lungs
   – Altered attenuation
   – Consolidation
   – Emphysema
   – Nodules and masses
   – Interstitium
● Airways
Mediastinal windows
● Pleura
● Mediastinum and hila
● Heart and vessels
   – Aorta
   – Pulmonary arteries
   – Heart and coronary vessels
● Soft tissues
● Below the diaphragm
Bone windows
● Bones

VENTILATION–PERFUSION ($\dot{V}/\dot{Q}$) SCAN

The primary role of $\dot{V}/\dot{Q}$ scanning is the identification of pulmonary embolism (PE). Lung perfusion scanning involves injection of microaggregates of albumin (MAA) labelled with the radionuclide technetium-99m. The MAA lodge within the pulmonary capillary bed and their distribution reflects regional lung perfusion. Ventilation images are acquired as the patient inhales a radioactive gas (e.g. krypton). Standard projections are posterior, anterior, and right and left posterior oblique. The two sets of images are scrutinized for perfusion defects in the absence of ventilation defects to confirm the presence of PE.

It is vital to understand the following terms when interpreting $\dot{V}/\dot{Q}$ scans: matched/mismatched defects and segmental/subsegmental and non-segmental defects.

❑ *Matched/mismatched defects*. A matched defect demonstrates ventilation *and* perfusion abnormalities of similar size in the same region. A mismatched defect displays reduced perfusion in an area of normal ventilation, or a much larger perfusion defect than ventilation abnormality (this is typical of PE).

45

Perfusion

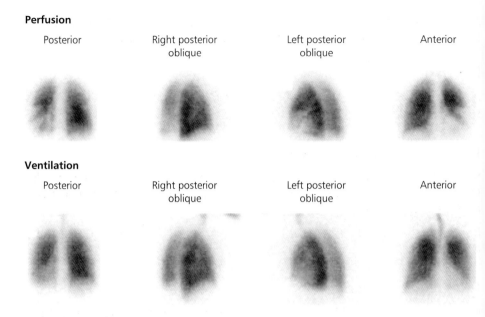

Fig. 3.9. Ventilation–perfusion scans. Note the wedge-shaped segmental perfusion defects involving the left lung. These extend to the pleural surface and are typical for pulmonary emboli. The defects are unmatched on the ventilation images.

❏ *Segmental/subsegmental/non-segmental defects.* Occlusion of a segmental branch of the pulmonary artery will lead to a subpleural, wedge-shaped, segmental perfusion defect (typical of PE). Sub-segmental perfusion defects are smaller than a whole segment. A non-segmental perfusion defect will not conform to segmental anatomy, and will not appear wedge shaped or subpleural.

Depending on the presence and number of perfusion defects, the $\dot{V}/\dot{Q}$ scan can be reported as normal, low, intermediate or high probability. These criteria were developed following a large US-based trial, the Prospective Investigation of Pulmonary Embolism Diagnosis (PIOPED) study.

Emboli are most commonly segmental; parenchymal disease is non-segmental; and sub-segmental defects are due to either emboli or parenchymal disease.

The typical appearances of PE on $\dot{V}/\dot{Q}$ scanning are shown in Fig. 3.9.

Clinical information

When looking for PE it is particularly important to determine its clinical likelihood.

Chest radiograph

Appraise this at the same time as the $\dot{V}/\dot{Q}$ scan. Lung parenchymal abnormalities, whether due to PE or another pathology, render the $\dot{V}/\dot{Q}$ more difficult to interpret.

A prominent aortic arch and hila, cardiomegaly, infection, pleural effusion and collapse may explain some unexpected appearances on the $\dot{V}/\dot{Q}$ scan.

Identify perfusion defects

Are these segmental/subsegmental (wedge shaped, subpleural) or are they non-segmental? The former strongly favour PE.

Identify ventilation defects

Segmental/subsegmental perfusion defects with normal ventilation indicate PE. Matched ventilation–perfusion defects or isolated ventilation defects alone point to a different pathology.

Beware that established PE can cause consolidation secondary to lung infarction and give a matched $\dot{V}/\dot{Q}$ defect.

Correlate findings

List the number, size and location of $\dot{V}/\dot{Q}$ mismatches and refer back to the chest radiograph. Discrete perfusion defects that are not explained by the chest radiograph are likely candidates for PE and, the greater the number of these defects, the higher is the probability of PE.

Interpretation Tips

Ventilation–perfusion scans

- Identify defects on two views to avoid over-calling PE.
- The ventilation scan can be differentiated from the perfusion scan by the presence of the trachea, which will also delineate anterior and posterior.
- When looking at the oblique projection, evaluate only the lung on that side.
- Subtly reduced, but not absent, perfusion can indicate a non-occlusive thrombus.
- If the scan is either normal or shows convincing evidence of PE, do not leave the clinicians in doubt of your diagnosis; however, do not be reticent in advising further imaging (i.e. CT pulmonary angiography) if it is inconclusive.

QUICK REFERENCE CHECKLIST

Clinical information
Review chest radiograph
Perfusion defects
Ventilation defects
Correlate findings
Probability of PE

MAMMOGRAPHY

The mammogram is the breast imaging investigation of choice in women aged over 35. Indications include the investigation of symptomatic breast lumps, breast cancer screening and follow-up after treatment for breast cancer.

Mediolateral oblique (MLO) and craniocaudal (CC) views of both breasts are acquired. During viewing these images should be placed side by side, along with any previous images, on a high-quality light box. A magnifying glass is used to aid viewing.

MAMMOGRAM

Technical factors

It is important that:

- ❏ the exposure is adequate and there is no movement blur.
- ❏ the MLO includes the lower axilla, the inframammary fold and the pectoral muscle down to the level of the nipple (Fig. 4.1)
- ❏ the CC view includes the retromammary space (i.e. the region of fat density posterior to the glandular tissue).

Background breast tissue

Comment on the background breast tissue. Younger patients tend to have more glandular (opaque) tissue, whereas older patients display more fatty (lucent) tissue.

Initial review

Scan the image for obvious focal lesions, noting any asymmetrical density, before performing a more thorough systematic review.

Systematic review

A suggested method for viewing the mammogram is to use a piece of card (e.g. the film packet) to sequentially block out parts of the images on both the right and left breasts simultaneously, thereby facilitating a comparison of small areas of breast tissue for asymmetry. This method was described by the charismatic Swedish radiologist Laszlo Tabar and is widely used to this day.

Fig. 4.1. Normal MLO (upper images) and CC (lower images) views of rather fatty breasts. The right MLO view is technically adequate, but the left view does not include the infra-mammary fold and the pectoral muscle does not extend down to the level of the nipple.

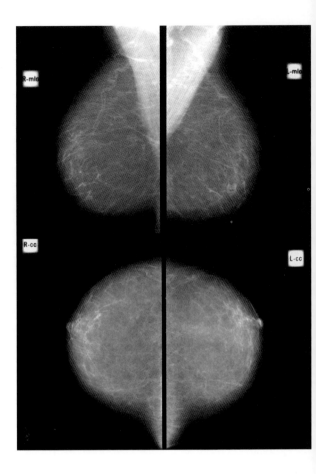

Closely analyse any abnormalities identified on systematic review and describe the following:

❏ *Site*. Give the location in terms of quadrants (the upper outer quadrant being the most common site of carcinoma).
❏ *Shape*. Rounded, oval or lobulated masses are generally benign. Irregular masses suggest malignancy.
❏ *Borders*. Well-defined borders usually indicate a benign lesion, whereas ill-defined, microlobulated or spiculated margins suggest malignancy.
❏ *Calcification*. If calcification is present, note whether it is punctate, curvilinear and well defined, with particles of a similar size and density (all these features indicate a benign process). Malignant calcification tends to have a 'crushed stone' appearance, with particles varying in size, shape and density. Linear, branching calcification should also raise suspicion.
❏ *Architectural distortion*. Carcinoma may masquerade as an area of subtle architectural distortion without a discernible mass.

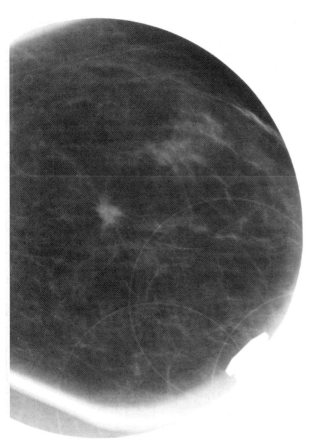

Fig. 4.2. Magnified paddle view of a typical spiculated carcinoma.

❏ *Asymmetrical density*. Focal differences in density between the breasts may be the only sign of cancer.
❏ *Associated features*. Look for additional signs of malignancy, such as enlarged axillary lymph nodes, vascular engorgement, abnormal ducts, nipple changes and skin thickening. Fig. 4.2 demonstrates a typical carcinoma.

Review areas

It is important to take a second look at the following areas, where pathology can easily be missed:

❏ behind the nipple in the area of dense glandular tissue (MLO and CC views)
❏ the 'Milky Way' – that is, the lucent, fat-rich part of the breast anterior to the pectoral muscles on the MLO and posterior on the CC
❏ the inframammary fold on the MLO.

Interpretation Tips

Mammogram

- If an abnormal area is identified, compression (paddle) views can be acquired with magnification to enhance detail.
- Give an overall assessment of whether a lesion is likely to be benign or malignant and decide on the need for further investigation (e.g. ultrasound, MRI and/or biopsy).
- Look for a lesion on two separate views (MLO and CC), but be aware that a lesion seen on only one view may be malignant.
- Raised skin lesions will be very clearly demarcated, as they are surrounded by air.

QUICK REFERENCE CHECKLIST

Mammogram

Technical factors
Background breast tissue
Initial review
Systematic review
- Site
- Shape
- Borders
- Calcification
- Architectural distortion
- Asymmetrical density
- Associated features
Review areas

ABDOMINAL RADIOLOGY 5

ABDOMINAL RADIOGRAPH

Technical factors

The abdominal film should include the lung bases and the groin hernial orifices, and should cover the properitoneal fat planes laterally.

Gastrointestinal gas pattern

Evaluate the intestinal gas pattern. On the normal abdominal film, a variable amount of gas may be seen within the stomach and the small and large bowel.

Colon

The colon usually occupies a peripheral location and contains faeces and gas. The haustra do not traverse the lumen, although the presence of overlapping haustra can sometimes give this impression. The maximal colonic diameter is said to be 8 cm, although this should be interpreted in the clinical context.

The caecal pole should be identified within the right iliac fossa. Its absence suggests malrotation, the caecum lying on a mesentery or, in the presence of small-bowel dilatation, a caecal volvulus.

Small bowel

In the normal patient, the small intestine is usually collapsed, and contains fluid and little gas. It may be appreciated only by the presence of small, irregular pockets of gas in a central location. Gas-filled small bowel is differentiated from the large bowel by its central location and the presence of the plicae circulares, which cross the lumen.

Note any thickening ('thumb-printing') of the bowel wall, which may be seen in inflammatory bowel disease (Fig. 5.1).

Abnormal gas

Intestinal obstruction

Small-bowel obstruction
Multiple, clearly discernible loops in the small bowel can indicate an obstruction, even if the small bowel is not excessively dilated. Small-bowel obstruction is not

Fig. 5.1. 'Thumb-printing' due to colitis – abnormal gas pattern within the transverse colon outlining oedematous mucosal folds (a).

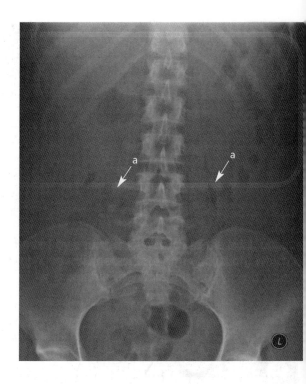

easily identified when the bowel loops are filled with fluid. In this situation, small amounts of gas will rise to the surface, and be visible on the supine radiograph as the 'string of beads' sign.

Occasionally, the cause of small-bowel obstruction may be seen:

❑ abnormal gas within the hernial orifices (incarcerated hernias)
❑ surgical clips indicating adhesions (Fig. 5.2)
❑ gallstone ileus.

Gallstone ileus is suggested by small-bowel obstruction and gas within the biliary tree. Occasionally a calcified gallstone may be seen.

Large-bowel obstruction
Identify whether a 'closed-loop' obstruction is present or whether the large bowel has decompressed into the small bowel through an incompetent ileocaecal valve.

Pneumoperitoneum

Signs can be subtle, particularly when the amount of gas is small. Signs to look for include the following:

❑ *The double wall* (Rigler's sign). The bowel wall is clearly discernible due to the presence of gas on both sides (Fig. 5.3).

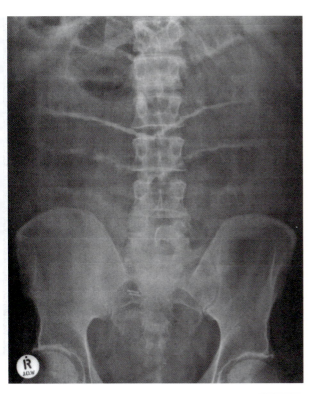

Fig. 5.2. Distended loops of centrally located, gas-filled bowel indicate small-bowel obstruction. The surgical clips within the pelvis raise the possibility of adhesions.

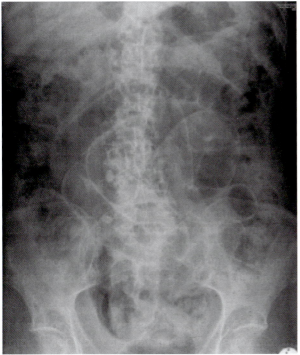

Fig. 5.3. Perforated duodenal ulcer and associated ileus. Note how both sides of the wall of the dilated small bowel are visible, signifying extraluminal as well as intraluminal gas – Rigler's sign.

❑ *Triangles of gas*. Look for small triangular or rhomboidal collections of gas lying between adjacent bowel loops.
❑ *Free air in the hepatorenal recess* (Morrison's pouch).
❑ *Football sign*. Larger collections of air may collect anterior to the abdominal viscera, giving rise to an ovoid, football-shaped radiolucency.
❑ *Retropneumoperitoneum*. Gas outlines the psoas muscles and kidneys.
❑ Gas may also outline the falciform and medial and lateral umbilical ligaments, or track into the fissure of ligamentum teres.

Other causes of abnormal gas

Other points to check include:

❑ portal venous gas (small branching gas lucency at the liver periphery) and gas in the bowel wall – both adverse signs
❑ gas within the urinary tract – secondary to a fistula or after instrumentation
❑ gas in the gallbladder wall – emphysematous cholecystitis.

Solid organs

Usually the liver, kidneys and spleen can be seen on the abdominal film. The size and shape of the liver are extremely variable and can extend down to the iliac crest (Riedel's lobe).

Fat and soft tissue

Usually a thin layer of extraperitoneal fat can be seen as lucency in both flanks – the properitoneal fat stripe. An accumulation of fluid in the paracolic gutters may lead to an increase in the width of the fluid density between the pro-peritoneal fat stripe and the colon.

Look for the outline of the psoas muscles diverging inferolaterally from the transverse processes of the lumbar vertebrae. Occasionally their absence may be suggestive of fluid or haemorrhage within the retroperitoneum, for example from a leaking aortic aneurysm or renal trauma (Fig. 5.4).

Calcification

Look for evidence of pathological intra-abdominal calcification (Table 5.1).

Bones

Do not neglect to look for bone pathology.

Foreign bodies

Check for lines, clips, joint prostheses, stents and so on.

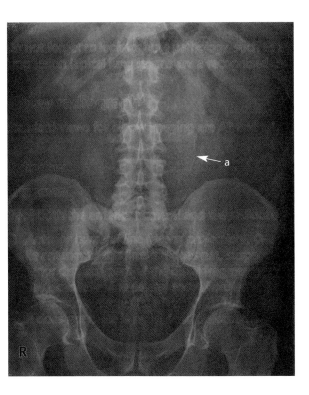

Fig. 5.4. Always check for an aortic aneurysm (a). In this case loss of definition of the left psoas muscle, in the context of acute abdominal pain, strongly suggests a retroperitoneal leak.

Table 5.1. Pathological intra-abdominal calcification

Site/type	Comment/appearance
Gallbladder	10% of gallstones calcify
Ureteric and bladder calculi	80% of ureteric calculi are radio-opaque
Vascular	
Abdominal aorta	Aneurysms may calcify
Splenic artery	
Phleboliths	Smooth, sub-5 mm, ovoid opacities, with or without a lucent centre, lying in the pelvis
Visceral	
Kidneys	May indicate renal calculi or intrinsic renal disease
Pancreas	Scattered calcification crossing the midline obliquely at L1
Prostate	Punctate calcification, relatively common
Lymph nodes	'Popcorn' calcification
Uterus	Fibroids often calcify
Adrenals	The adrenals are usually seen only if calcified; calcification is often bilateral

Interpretation Tips

Abdominal radiograph

● Commonly missed pathology/review areas include groin hernias, abdominal aortic aneurysms (as they are projected over the spine) and subtle pneumoperitoneum.
● A caecal diameter of greater than 9 cm with clinical caecal tenderness is a sign of imminent perforation.
● Psoas shadows are not seen under normal circumstances in a significant proportion of patients.
● Ankylosing spondylitis and sacroileitis may be present in individuals with inflammatory bowel disease.

QUICK REFERENCE CHECKLIST

Abdominal radiograph

Technical factors
Gastrointestinal gas pattern
● Colon
● Small bowel
Abnormal gas
● Intestinal obstruction
● Pneumoperitoneum
● Other causes of abnormal gas
Solid organs
Fat and soft tissue
Calcification
Bones
Foreign bodies

INTRAVENOUS UROGRAM (IVU)

The most common indication for the IVU is renal stone disease, although it is being replaced by unenhanced CT in some centres. Other indications include haematuria, renal tract trauma and recurrent urinary tract infection. The following system is weighted towards the IVU performed for renal colic secondary to calculus disease.

There is no set series of post-contrast images. The IVU should be viewed as a dynamic process with extra images tailored to answer the question posed. A balance needs to be struck between radiation protection (fewer films) and the acquisition of sufficient images to secure a diagnosis. Often, with classic renal colic, a control film and a single, full-length, delayed (15- to 20-minute) post-micturition film can elucidate the cause and level of obstruction. Supplementary investigation with ultrasound or CT may be warranted, dependent on the IVU findings. Fig. 5.5 shows an example of ureteric obstruction on IVU.

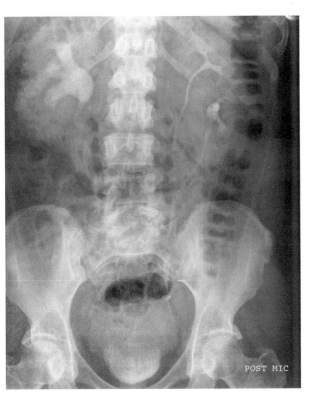

Fig. 5.5. Full-length, post-micturition radiograph demonstrating an obstructed right-sided system, in this case due to a calculus at the right vesicoureteric junction. There is an unobstructed left-sided duplex kidney with ureteric duplication. In addition, note the lumbar spinal closure abnormality.

Pre-contrast control film

Appraise as for any abdominal radiograph (see pp. 53–58). In particular, pay close attention to calcification that may be obscured later by contrast. Common causes of urinary tract calcification are urinary tract calculi, nephrocalcinosis, localized calcification due to conditions such as tuberculosis and prostatic calcification. Oblique views can help determine whether calcification is within, or projected over, the renal tract.

Post-contrast film

Renal position

The left kidney usually lies above the right. The axis lies parallel to the outer margins of the psoas muscles. Abnormal renal position can be the result of congenital malposition, or due to a displacing retroperitoneal mass.

Renal size, shape and outline

The normal kidney is 9–13 cm in length. Although the left kidney is often slightly larger than the right, a difference in length of over 1.5 cm should raise suspicion of a duplex system in the larger kidney, or scarring of the smaller kidney. The outlines are normally smooth, and indentations (e.g. cortical scarring) or bulges (e.g. masses) must be explained. The left kidney often displays a 'splenic hump' in the interpolar region as a normal variant. The parenchymal width should be uniform. If a mass is present, look to see if underlying calyces are distorted.

The presence of a duplex system or horseshoe kidney should be apparent.

Calyces

These should be well filled, evenly distributed and reasonably symmetrical. The outer margins should be cup shaped. Dilatation of the calyces causes a blunted or clubbed appearance. Calyceal dilatation is most commonly caused by obstruction, but bear in mind that destruction of the papilla (e.g. chronic pyelonephritis) will give a similar appearance. Obstruction may be unilateral (e.g. calculus disease) or bilateral (e.g. bladder outflow obstruction caused by prostatic hypertrophy). Look for contrast leaching out into the surrounding perirenal space, which can occur with complete ureteric obstruction. Look for filling defects within the calyces, but beware of vascular impressions falsely suggesting filling defects.

Pelvis

Calyceal dilatation is invariably accompanied by a degree of pelvic dilatation in obstruction. Compare with the contralateral side. A dilated pelvis in the absence of calyceal dilatation probably represents an extrarenal pelvis, which is a normal variant. Filling defects can be caused by calculi, tumour or clot.

Ureters

Look for ureteric dilatation and identify the level if obstruction is present. Normal ureters are rarely seen in their full length, because of peristaltic contractions, so a dilated ureter with a standing column of contrast indicates obstruction. Check ureteric alignment, as retroperitoneal masses can cause ureteric displacement.

Bladder

If a pre-micturition film has been acquired, assess shape, size and outline of the bladder. An enlarged prostate may be apparent, indenting the bladder. Following micturition, the bladder should empty almost completely. Filling defects warrant further investigation.

Interpretation Tips

IVU

- A delay in contrast excretion suggests obstruction. A delayed image should be left approximately three to four times longer than the previous image (this should be taken as a rough guide and each case should be judged individually).
- Renal tomography is useful if bowel gas overlies the kidneys, making contrast detail difficult to define.
- In the absence of obstruction, consider compression or scanning the patient prone or in the Trendelenburg position to distend the ureters and calyces fully.
- The passage of a calculus can lead to oedema within the vesicoureteric junction, which in turn will lead to mild residual dilatation of the ureter and pelvicalyceal system on that side.
- Increased loin pain shortly after contrast injection often occurs if there is genuine obstruction.
- Obstruction may not cause gross pelvicalyceal dilatation if contrast leaches out of the calyces into the perirenal space (this may also cause pain).
- Leaking aortic aneurysms may mimic renal colic; therefore, look at the rest of the abdomen on the IVU series for relevant clues as to the patient's presentation.

QUICK REFERENCE CHECKLIST

IVU

Pre-contrast
- Control film

Post-contrast
- Renal position
- Renal size, shape and outline
- Calyces
- Pelvis
- Ureters
- Bladder

CONTRAST SWALLOW

Although endoscopy has largely replaced the contrast swallow, it still plays a valuable role in the diagnosis of oesophageal pathology, as it provides both functional and anatomical information. Barium is the contrast of choice; however, if aspiration or an oesophageal leak/perforation is suspected, water-soluble contrast such as Gastromiro should be used. Better oesophageal mucosal detail is provided if effervescent granules (e.g. Carbex) are given before the study (double contrast).

Oropharynx

Check that swallowing initiates normally. Look for pooling of contrast within the mouth and reflux into the nasopharynx. Abnormalities in the initiation of swallowing indicate bulbar pathology.

Aspiration

On the lateral view, look for contrast passing anteriorly into the laryngeal vestibule, termed 'penetration'. Passage through the vocal cords signifies aspiration.

Pharyngeal pouch

Diverticula can arise along the length of the oesophagus. Specifically look for a pharyngeal pouch – a diverticulum arising due to weakness of the pharyngeal muscles posterior to the proximal oesophagus.

Web

Look for a sharp indentation within the anterior proximal oesophagus.

Leaks

Following oesophageal surgery look carefully for anastomotic leak.

Motility

Assess overall oesophageal motility marked by a smooth peristaltic stripping wave. Uncoordinated contractions cause a rippled, undulating oesophageal appearance, termed 'tertiary contractions' or 'corkscrew oesophagus'.

Oesophageal mucosa

The mucosa should be smooth with longitudinal folds. Identify ulcers within the mucosa, or any irregularity of the wall – a 'cobblestone' pattern – which may indicate oesophageal candidiasis in immunocompromised individuals.

Strictures

Strictures should always raise the spectre of malignancy. Assess the overall length, shape and location of a stricture to provide a clue to the aetiology:

- ❏ carcinoma – irregular, circumferential, shouldering, over several centimetres, with or without a soft-tissue mass (Fig. 5.6)
- ❏ peptic – distal oesophagus, short, smooth outlines, tapered (not shouldered) edges, often associated with hiatus hernia.

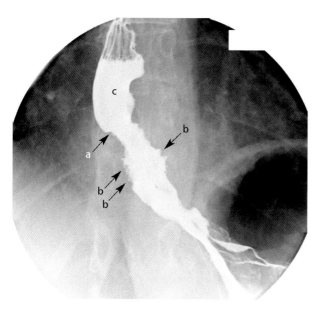

Fig. 5.6. Barium swallow demonstrating shouldering (a), mucosal irregularity and small ulcer pits (b). There is also hold-up of contrast within the distal oesophagus (c). These features are typical of a distal oesophageal cancer.

Other types of stricture include post-corrosive ingestion (long stricture) and achalasia (smooth narrowing of the distal oesophagus with proximal dilatation and food residue).

Filling defects

These may be intraluminal (e.g. food bolus), intramural (e.g. tumour) or extrinsic (e.g. bronchial carcinoma). Beware of the normal impression of the aortic arch and left main bronchus. Lucent, serpiginous filling defects indicate varices.

Dilatation

Dilatation may be the result of a distal obstructing lesion (e.g. carcinoma) or a systemic disorder (e.g. scleroderma).

Position of the gastro-oesophageal junction

Identify the relation of the gastro-oesophageal junction to the diaphragm. If a hiatus hernia is identified, decide whether it is sliding or rolling.

Stomach

Although the primary aim of the contrast swallow is to evaluate the oesophagus, views of the stomach may reveal an obvious filling defect or ulcerating lesion.

Image periphery

Review the extra-oesophageal structures on the images in case an incidental lung carcinoma or vertebral lesion is evident.

Interpretation Tips

Contrast swallow

- For solid food dysphagia or dysmotility, consider giving a semi-solid bolus (barium-soaked marshmallow or bread).
- If stomach pathology is suspected, early stomach views are indicated, as duodenal flooding with contrast can obscure the stomach.
- A right anterior oblique view gives the clearest oesophageal detail, as it is projected off the vertebral column.
- The prone swallow can accentuate reflux of gastric contents back into the oesophagus.

QUICK REFERENCE CHECKLIST

Contrast swallow

Oropharynx
Aspiration
Pharyngeal pouch
Web
Leaks
Motility
Oesophageal mucosa
Strictures
Filling defects
Dilatation
Position of the gastro-oesophageal junction
Stomach
Image periphery

SMALL-BOWEL CONTRAST STUDY

Barium is the contrast of choice for small-bowel studies of the jejunum and ileum. (The stomach and duodenum are best assessed with either endoscopy or barium meal.)

The small bowel can be studied after ingestion of an oral contrast medium – small-bowel follow-through – or following injection of the contrast medium into the proximal jejunum via a nasojejunal tube – small-bowel enema (enteroclysis).

Particular attention should be paid to the terminal ileum, as this is a common site of small-bowel pathology. The investigation of Crohn's disease (CD) is the commonest indication for this study.

Barium transit

Comment on the overall transit time, noting any hold-up to the free passage of the contrast medium.

Position and mobility of the small bowel

Note any abnormality of the position of the small bowel. It may be displaced by masses, or located in an abnormal position secondary to congenital malrotation. Bowel loops should be mobile on palpation.

Luminal narrowing

This may be due to the following:

❏ *Normal peristalsis*. This produces transient, smooth concentric narrowing, with preservation of mucosal folds
❏ *Strictures*. These are seen as permanent, irregular narrowing with loss of mucosal folds, often with proximal dilatation (Fig. 5.7).
❏ *Extrinsic compression*. Only one wall is compressed and bowel loops may be displaced by the mass.
❏ *Adhesions*. These are difficult to diagnose on a contrast study but may be suggested by apparent tethering of bowel loops or evidence of previous surgery.

Dilatation

Identify areas of dilatation (>3 cm ileum, >4 cm jejunum), which indicate potential obstruction, paralytic ileus or malabsorption.

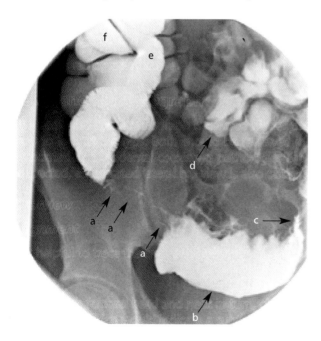

Fig. 5.7. Small-bowel follow-through, demonstrating distal ileal stricturing (a) and dilatation of the pre-anastomotic segment (b). Note that there is an apparent second stricture more proximally (c), with separation of the abnormal ileal segment from the normal small-bowel loops (d). These appearances are typical of small-bowel Crohn's disease. e = terminal ileum, f = caecum.

Mucosal pathology

Fold thickening

The normal fold thickness is <3 mm. Fold thickening is a non-specific sign indicating inflammation or infiltration of the bowel wall.

Mucosal ulceration

Normally the wall is smooth. Ulcers manifest as sharp, contrast-filled projections in the bowel wall. Ulceration occurs in CD, lymphoma and tuberculosis. Confluent ulceration, particularly at the terminal ileum, may give a 'cobblestone' appearance in CD.

Fistula formation

Look for abnormal passage of contrast medium between bowel and adjacent viscera.

Caecum

As contrast medium spills out into the large bowel, focus on the iliocaecal valve and caecum, and note any obvious lesions.

Outside the bowel

Do not forget to look for additional pathology that may be relevant (e.g. sacroileitis in inflammatory bowel disease).

Interpretation Tips

Small-bowel contrast study

● Palpate the bowel during the examination to separate loops of bowel, particularly around the terminal ileum, in order to render any pathology more clearly visible.
● Negative contrast (e.g. methylcellulose) can be given during a small-bowel enema to enhance mucosal detail.
● The presence of contrast medium within the large bowel before it reaches the terminal ileum indicates an enteroenteric fistula.

Small-bowel contrast study

Barium transit
Position and mobility of the small bowel
Luminal narrowing
Dilatation
Mucosal pathology
Caecum
Outside the bowel

DOUBLE-CONTRAST BARIUM ENEMA

Following bowel preparation, barium and air (or CO_2) are introduced into the colon to outline the mucosa in double contrast. The contrast medium should reach the caecum, marked by reflux into the appendix or terminal ileum. The length of the colon can vary considerably, as can the anatomical position of bowel loops, depending on the length of the mesentery. The barium enema is a dynamic study and it is important to recognize pathology as the examination progresses and to tailor it accordingly.

Luminal narrowing

Look for luminal narrowing and if present try to determine its cause: strictures, spasm or extrinsic compression.

Strictures

Causes include carcinoma, diverticular disease, ischaemic colitis, CD and radiation fibrosis. The site of a lesion provides a clue as to the origin. For example, diverticular strictures invariably involve the sigmoid colon. In CD, strictures affect the right-sided colon preferentially and may be multiple ('skip' lesions).

If a stricture is identified, then endoscopy and biopsy are indicated.

The typical differences between benign and malignant strictures are summarized in Table 5.2.

Table 5.2. The typical differences between benign and malignant strictures

	Length	Outline	Edges	Longitudinal folds
Benign stricture	Any length	Smooth outline	Tapered edges	Retained
Malignant stricture	Typically short	Irregular outline	Shouldered edges ('apple-core lesion')	Lost

Fig. 5.8. Double-contrast barium enema demonstrating a large splenic flexure carcinoma. Note the shouldering (a), stricturing (b), polypoid mass (c) and incidental diverticular disease (d).

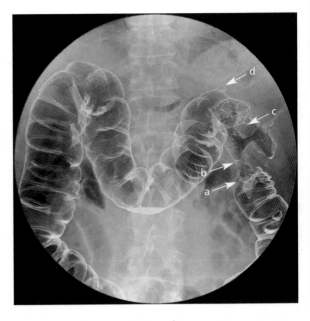

A malignant stricture is demonstrated in Fig. 5.8.

Spasm

The use of anti-spasmodics during the examination (Buscopan and glucagon) reduce spasm.

Look for smooth, concentric narrowing that is transient. Note that spasm can affect diseased bowel, masking pathology.

Extrinsic compression

Look for narrowing whereby one wall is compressed by an external mass.

Diverticula

Diverticula are very common spherical mucosal out-pouchings through a hypertrophied muscular bowel wall. They are commonest in the sigmoid but can occur throughout the colon. Inflammation (diverticulitis) may lead to stricture or fistula formation.

Filling defects

Polyps may be single or multiple, sessile or pedunculated. Features suggesting carcinoma are a thick stalk, an irregular surface and a diameter of over 2 cm. All polyps over 1 cm should be removed owing to the possibility of malignancy.

Faeces may mimic polyps, but are completely surrounded by barium and air with no attachment to the wall and move freely when seen on serial images.

Ulceration

The mucosa is normally smooth, and therefore sharp projections of contrast medium seen projecting into the wall of the bowel suggest ulceration (typical in inflammatory bowel disease).

Pre-sacral space and rectum

The pre-sacral space should be less then 1 cm at S4 when evaluated on the lateral view; more than this indicates pathology at this site. The rectal folds should be less than 5 mm thick; the fold thickness may be increased by tumour or inflammation.

Terminal ileum

If reflux of barium is seen within the terminal ileum, look for stricturing and irregularity typical of terminal ileal disease.

Interpretation Tips

Double-contrast barium enema

● Low rectal tumours can be missed with a double-contrast barium enema, as the rectal tube obscures them; therefore, per-rectum examination is indicated before the procedure.
● If one colonic carcinoma is seen, search hard for a second, as contiguous cancers are common.
● It may be difficult to distinguish a small polyp from a diverticulum. Try to get a view in profile in order to see if it protrudes into (polyp) or out of the lumen (diverticulum). In addition, when seen in double contrast *en face*, polyps have a sharply defined inner margin and diverticula sharply defined outer margin.

QUICK REFERENCE CHECKLIST

Double-contrast barium enema

Luminal narrowing
● Strictures
● Spasm
● Extrinsic compression
Diverticula
Filling defects
Ulceration
Pre-sacral space and rectum
Terminal ileum
Outside the bowel

Outside the bowel

Do not neglect to look at the periphery of the image for relevant pathology not directly related to the bowel (e.g. sacroileitis, gallstones). Large abdominal masses will displace bowel loops.

ABDOMINAL CT: OVERVIEW

The diagnostic information that can be gleaned from abdominal CT depends on the imaging protocol used. Bear the following in mind during interpretation:

❏ whether intravenous contrast has been used and the volume and rate of administration
❏ the phase of image acquisition following contrast administration
❏ the type of enteric contrast used (positive or negative), the route (e.g. nasogastric, oral, rectal) and the time of administration
❏ methods to promote bowel distension (e.g. drugs, air, osmotic contrast agents).

Things not to miss in the acute abdomen

It is important to note the presence of free intra-abdominal fluid, faeces and abnormal gas. Significant collections of fluid, faeces and gas can be surprisingly easy to miss. It is also important to check for changes to the bowel wall and intra-abdominal fat.

Free fluid

Free intraperitoneal fluid tends to accumulate in dependent areas, such as the pelvis, paracolic gutters and the root of the small-bowel mesentery, or in the peritoneal recesses, for example the subphrenic spaces and lesser sac. The nature of the fluid is difficult to ascertain on CT but the presence of gas or an enhancing rim raises the possibility of infection.

Faecal peritonitis

Free intraperitoneal faeces can be mistaken for a colonic loop, so check that all faeces are bounded by a bowel wall.

Abnormal gas

Small pockets of extraluminal gas are best appreciated on wider windows (e.g. lung windows). Do not forget gas accumulation in the wall of the bowel, or gas in the biliary tree, portal veins and soft tissues.

Bowel wall changes

These features are non-specific and are seen in many disease processes. Look for the following:

❑ *Wall thickening.*
❑ *Mural stratification.*
❑ *Accumulation of low-attenuation submucosal oedema or fat* (acute and chronic inflammation, respectively). Such accumulations can lead to a 'halo' appearance of the bowel wall. The differential here is wide and includes infective, inflammatory and ischaemic processes.
❑ *Mucosal enhancement.* Mucosal hyperenhancement is a characteristic finding in active inflammation (e.g. inflammatory bowel disease) and in ischaemic bowel. Absent, or poor, mucosal enhancement is seen in severe ischaemia.
❑ *Intramural gas.* In the appropriate clinical context, intramural gas can indicate disruption of bowel integrity and is a poor prognostic indicator.

Changes in intra-abdominal fat

Most individuals have sufficient intra-abdominal fat to identify the small- and large-bowel mesenteries. Increased density or stranding within the intra-abdominal fat is often the principal clue to disease in the underlying viscus. Its presence can signify intra-abdominal fat infiltrated by inflammatory cells, fluid, tumour or fibrosis.

Characterization of masses

CT is commonly employed in the characterization of masses and the staging of cancer. A thorough examination of the features of a mass can narrow the diagnosis, stage disease and aid treatment planning. Comment on:

❑ size and shape
❑ likely site of origin
❑ density (e.g. fat, fluid, soft tissue, calcification)
❑ borders (e.g. well defined or ill defined)
❑ cystic masses – wall thickening, nodularity, septation (fine septations may not be appreciated)
❑ effect on surrounding structures
❑ enhancement pattern – hypervascular or hypovascular
❑ vascular supply – note whether this is aberrant or unusual
❑ lymphadenopathy and metastases.

ABDOMINAL CT: SYSTEMATIC REVIEW OF ORGAN SYSTEMS

Liver and biliary tree

The systematic reviews of the liver and biliary tree are detailed separately below (see pages 80–84).

Bowel

The small intestine is usually best imaged using CT enterography techniques that make use of thin sections and large volumes of enteric contrast agent to display the small-bowel lumen and wall.

Beware of the following issues when evaluating pathology of the stomach and bowel:

❏ Poorly distended bowel segments (usually due to normal peristalsis) may simulate mural thickening and luminal narrowing, falsely suggesting inflammatory stricturing or tumour. Good bowel distension can be achieved with the use of anti-spasmodic agents and administration of adequate volumes of oral fluid. A large drink immediately prior to scanning is often advocated to promote adequate distension of the stomach and duodenum.

❏ Because of problems with inadequate distension, it is often difficult to diagnose pathology in the stomach. CT is primarily used as an adjunct to endoscopy, for staging a mass discovered at endoscopy or to direct endoscopic examination to an area of suspicion.

❏ Pathological mural enhancement may be obscured by intraluminal positive contrast agents and so negative contrast agents (e.g. water) are often preferred.

❏ Positive contrast agents may be preferred to obtain information on bowel transit in suspected intestinal obstruction.

Bowel wall changes

See above – 'Things not to miss in the acute abdomen' (page 70).

Bowel obstruction

The identification of dilated proximal and collapsed distal bowel, with an abrupt transition point between the two, is suggestive of bowel obstruction. Seek out the following features:

❏ *The level and site of the obstruction*. Do not forget to check hernial orifices. Internal hernias can be subtle and are suggested by an abnormal passage of vessels and mesentery through an apparent defect.

❏ *The small-bowel faeces sign*. This is a characteristic finding in small-bowel obstruction; it suggests prolonged stasis of intestinal content, which resembles colonic faecal residue. It is often greatest just proximal to the point of obstruction.

❏ *The presence of a closed loop obstruction*. A closed loop obstruction is defined as a mechanical obstruction at at least two points. This carries a worse prognosis than simple obstruction. It is suggested by: a cluster or segment of dilated bowel loops; a radial arrangement of the mesentery and vessels converging to a single point; mesenteric and vascular congestion.

Bowel cancer

Follow the entire length of the colon checking for a colorectal tumour as evidenced by the presence of a mass, stricture, peri-enteric changes, lymphadenopathy and metastases.

Interpretation Tips

CT of the bowel

● Unless dedicated CT colonography is performed, usually only large colonic masses may be appreciated.
● Three-dimensional multiplanar reformats can aid in visualization of the transitional point of bowel obstruction.

Pancreas

Imaging protocols vary between departments, but up to three phases (unenhanced, arterial and portal venous phases) of image acquisition may be necessary for full evaluation. Large volumes of contrast medium at high flow rates lead to greater enhancement of normal parenchyma and increase the conspicuousness of pathological changes.

CT is primarily used in the identification and assessment of pancreatic masses and the evaluation of inflammatory diseases of the pancreas. The imaging features that need to be evaluated in these conditions are summarized below.

Acute pancreatitis

This is suggested by:

❏ biliary calculi and obstruction
❏ diffuse or focal pancreatic enlargement
❏ increased attenuation and stranding of the peripancreatic fat (poor pancreatic enhancement is taken as an indicator of glandular necrosis, the degree of which should be estimated)
❏ peripancreatic and intra-abdominal fluid collections (the presence of gas pockets within these suggests either an infected collection or bowel fistulation, both adverse prognostic features)
❏ vascular complications, including venous thrombosis (splenic, mesenteric and portal veins), collateral formation, portal hypertension, and arterial pseudoaneurysm formation.

Chronic pancreatitis

Chronic pancreatitis is suggested by:

❏ glandular atrophy and calcification
❏ ductal calculi
❏ foci of active inflammation.

Focal pancreatic masses

Pancreatic adenocarcinoma

Pancreatic adenocarcinoma is an ill-defined, poorly enhancing pancreatic mass. Sometimes the presence of a mass can be inferred if dilatation of both the pancreatic and common bile ducts is present. Assess for the presence of vascular encasement and nodal and visceral metastases.

Neuroendocrine cell tumours
These appear as avidly enhancing small tumours.

Cystic lesions
Mucinous and serous pancreatic tumours often have characteristic patterns of calcification. True benign pancreatic cysts are unusual.

Intraductal papillary mucinous tumours
These are primarily cystic lesions with variable malignant potential.

Interpretation Tips

CT of the pancreas

● Pancreatic enhancement can be decreased in normal patients with fatty infiltration of the pancreas.
● There may be variation in pancreatic enhancement between the head and the tail (<30 HU), which should not be confused with glandular necrosis.
● As glandular necrosis develops at around 72 hours, CT performed after 3 days yields higher accuracy in diagnosing necrotizing pancreatitis.
● Focal inflammation may be indistinguishable from a pancreatic tumour.

Urinary tract

Common indications for CT include renal colic, mass lesions, trauma and renal angiography.

Five distinct phases of renal contrast enhancement are described.

❏ renal arterial enhancement, at 10–25 s
❏ renal cortical enhancement, the corticomedullary phase, at 40–70 s
❏ equal enhancement of the cortex and medulla, the nephrographic phase, at 80–100 s
❏ presence of contrast in the calyces and pelvis, the excretory phase, at 120 s
❏ delayed scans performed at 5–10 min to visualize the ureters and bladder.

General assessment of the urinary tract

Check for the following:

❏ congenital malformations and anatomical variants
❏ renal size
❏ contour – an irregular contour may result from renal scarring or a mass

❏ cortical thickness – diffuse thinning of the cortex suggests a chronic renal insult
❏ pelvicalyceal dilatation and clubbing
❏ ureteric malformations – duplications, ectopic insertions, abnormal course
❏ mass lesions (see under Characterization of masses', p. 71).

Renal colic

Identify the site and size of ureteric calculi. Calculi tend to lodge at the pelviureteric junction, the pelvic brim or the vesicoureteric junction.

Confirm that the calculus lies within the ureter. Look for periureteric fat stranding.

Seek out signs of ureteric obstruction:

❏ proximal ureteric dilatation and hydronephrosis
❏ renal enlargement
❏ perinephric stranding
❏ periureteric stranding.

Poor enhancement of the affected kidney indicates a secondary reduction in its perfusion.

Interpretation Tips

CT of the urinary tract

● Positive oral contrast may obscure renal calculi if opacified bowel lies nearby.
● An unenhanced scan can be performed initially to look for radio-opaque calculi.
● It is not always possible to ascertain whether a radio-opaque calcification represents a ureteric calculus, a phlebolith or vascular calcification. Intravenous contrast (CT urography) is warranted in these cases to outline the ureter.
● If a calculus appears lodged in the distal ureter at the ureterovesical junction when the patient is supine, this can be differentiated from a calculus lying dependently in the bladder by turning the patient prone and rescanning.
● A dilated, non-obstructed, extra-renal pelvis can simulate an obstruction at the pelviureteric junction; however, there will be no associated calyceal dilatation.
● Where there are cystic renal masses, look for wall thickening, calcification, size, internal complexity and enhancement.
● In suspected urothelial tumour, a delayed scan will permit assessment of filling defects (e.g. transitional cell carcinoma) within the ureters and collecting system.

Adrenals

The discovery of an incidental adrenal mass occurs in up to 5% of abdominal CT examinations. Note the following:

❏ *Size*. Most nodules under 3 cm are benign; the likelihood of malignancy rises above this size.

❏ *Density*. Adenomas tend to be low density, secondary to the presence of intra-cellular lipid.
❏ *Washout characteristics*. All adenomas tend to have a more rapid loss of atten-uation value soon after enhancement with contrast material than malignant lesions.

Interpretation Tip

CT of the adrenals

● An adrenal mass even in a patient with a known malignancy is not always a metas-tasis.

Spleen

The spleen is evaluated best on portal venous imaging, as its appearance on the arterial phase is variable, owing to differential perfusion of the red and white pulp.

Comment on:

❏ size – atrophy or enlargement
❏ focal lesions within the spleen
❏ spleniculi (these well-rounded soft-tissue nodules in the vicinity of the spleen display the same enhancement characteristics as the spleen).

Lymph nodes

Malignant neoplasms initially spread to their local or regional draining lymph node groups, but, with more advanced disease, other lymph node groups may become involved. Involvement can lead to enlargement and it is this that the radiologist is looking for.

Some diseases, notably lymphoma, can result in widespread adenopathy, albeit often in characteristic sites. Knowledge of lymph drainage will allow the radiologist to evaluate specifically those areas likely to be associated with a particular malignant disease. Generally, lymph drainage corresponds to the vascular supply of the given organ. Unfortunately, CT is notoriously insensitive in identifying the presence of tumour in a lymph node. Nodal enlargement in the abdomen, as elsewhere, can be the result of infection. It is often a combination of features that suggests patho-logical lymph node enlargement:

❏ *Size*. Lymph nodes are measured in their short axis by convention and greater than 1 cm is often considered pathological. However this is neither sensitive nor specific for tumour.
❏ *Number*. A cluster of lymph nodes in a particular drainage territory may suggest malignancy, particularly when they are enlarged.
❏ *Density*. Nodes with a central low density imply the presence of necrosis and are nearly always pathological.

❏ *Confluent lymph nodes*. Lymph node masses encasing or displacing vessels are seen in neoplasia, particularly lymphoma.

Vessels

Major vessels are best evaluated by threshold-triggered scanning, especially when assessing the arterial system. Look at the arteries and check for aneurysms.

Arteries

Look for:

❏ mural thrombosis
❏ intimal calcification
❏ evidence of end-organ ischaemia (e.g. differential renal enhancement, mesenteric ischaemia).

Aneurysms

Check the following:

❏ proximal and distal extent
❏ whether fusiform or saccular
❏ peri-arterial soft-tissue stranding (implies inflammatory aetiology)
❏ evidence of leak.

Veins

Look for:

❏ occlusive venous thrombosis (IVC, portal vein).

Pelvis

The evaluation of the pelvis can be challenging on CT, because of the lack of soft-tissue contrast, and MRI is often preferred. The use of rectally administered contrast can considerably aid interpretation. Rarely the vagina needs to be outlined; a tampon is usually simplest.

Anatomical considerations

The ovaries are intraperitoneal, therefore spread of ovarian carcinoma is commonly intraperitoneal. In contrast, the uterus and cervix lie beneath the peritoneal reflection. The uterus, cervix and upper vagina are related on their lateral surface to the parametrium, which extends laterally toward the pelvic sidewalls. The parametria usually have no definable margins on CT because the broad ligament, which marks their anatomical boundaries, is not seen.

Ovaries

The general criteria for radiological assessment of masses apply here. When assessing predominantly cystic masses, pay particular attention to the presence of septation, calcification and enhancing soft-tissue components. Ultrasound and MRI have complementary roles.

Uterus and cervix

When assessing masses of the uterus and cervix, check for involvement of the para-metrium, as this signifies local disease spread. Again, MRI is the preferred modal-ity. Involvement of the pelvic sidewall is suggested by masses spreading to the internal iliac lymphovascular structures and the obturator internus or piriformis muscles. Look for ureteric obstruction leading to hydronephrosis. Do not forget to look for posterior extension into the perirectal fat.

Prostate

CT is generally not used for local staging of prostate cancer, although occasionally an asymmetric mass in the prostate may be appreciated.

Rectum and sigmoid colon

MRI is preferred for staging rectal carcinoma but CT may detect sigmoid and rectal tumours incidentally. Look for tumour spread and nodularity in the adjacent fat. This is relatively well seen around the rectum in most patients.

Sigmoid diverticulosis is extremely common, as are complications from this, such as inflammation (diverticulitis), abscess formation, perforation and fistulation. These should all be looked for routinely. Do not forget that a tumour can also give rise to these complications.

Bones

Switch to bone windows and look in sagittal, coronal and axial planes to aid visu-alization of bone lesions. For example, widespread prostatic bony metastases (Fig. 5.9) are not as readily apparent until viewed on dedicated bone windows (Fig. 5.10).

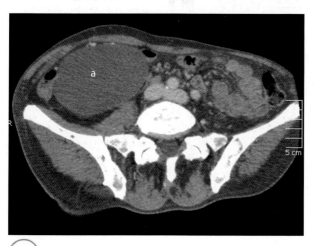

Fig. 5.9. Widespread prostatic bony metastases are not as readily apparent until viewed on dedicated bone windows (Fig. 5.10). The original indication for this abdominal window scan was to assess the size of the large cyst arising from the lower pole of the right kidney (a).

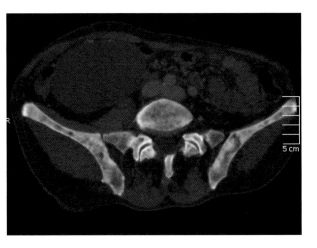

Fig. 5.10. Widespread prostatic bony metastases more readily apparent viewed on dedicated bone windows.

Remember that inflammatory bowel disease is associated with arthropathy of the axial skeleton, in particular the sacroiliac joints.

Review areas

❑ *Peritoneum and omentum.* Peritoneal and omental nodularity and thickening usually occur as a result of neoplasia or occasionally inflammatory or infective processes.
❑ *Lung bases.*
❑ *Foreign bodies (drains, stents, clips, catheters, etc.).* Comment on the adequacy of positioning and confirm with contrast if necessary.

Systematic review can elucidate a unifying diagnosis in abdominal imaging with CT (Fig. 5.11).

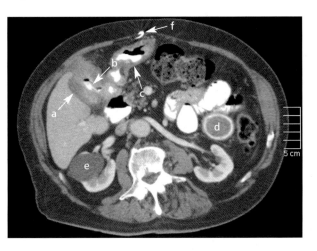

Fig. 5.11. Axial image through the abdomen showing a thick-walled gallbladder (a), with surrounding inflammatory change. Oral contrast and gas are seen within the gallbladder (b), indicating a fistula to the thick-walled proximal duodenum (c). The fistula was formed by a large gallstone that eroded through the gallbladder wall into the small bowel, which now rests within the proximal jejunum (d). Incidental note is made of a right renal cyst (e) and surgical clips (f).

Abdominal CT

Things not to miss:
● Free fluid
● Faecal peritonitis
● Abnormal gas
● Bowel wall changes
● Intra-abdominal fat stranding
Liver and biliary tree
Bowel
Pancreas
Urinary tract
Adrenal glands
Spleen
Lymph nodes
Vessels
Pelvis
Bones
Review areas

ABDOMINAL CT: SYSTEMATIC REVIEW OF THE LIVER AND BILIARY TREE

Advances in liver imaging have resulted in a general trend towards definitive image-guided diagnosis and away from percutaneous biopsy. The radiologist is increasingly being asked to identify those lesions that can be left well alone and those that require surgical resection.

Liver perfusion

Understanding the perfusion of the liver is central to understanding the different imaging appearances. The liver has a dual blood supply, comprising inflow from the hepatic portal vein of 1000–1200 ml/min and from the hepatic artery at 400 ml/min.

Phase of image acquisition and technical adequacy

The liver can vary widely in appearance, depending on the timing of image acquisition after contrast injection. It is possible to overlook significant pathology if either the acquisition is inappropriately timed or a small quantity of contrast is given too slowly, resulting in mixing of the arterial and portal venous phases of liver perfusion. Figs 7.12 and 7.13 show the importance of dual phase imaging in abdominal CT. They are two axial images at the same level. The arterial phase image (Fig. 5.12)

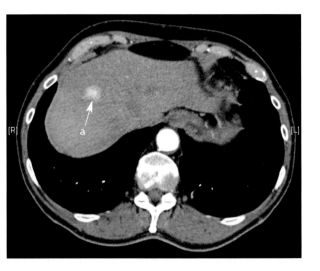

Fig. 5.12. Arterial phase image clearly demonstrating a hypervascular lesion (a).

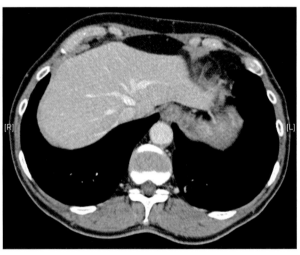

Fig. 5.13. Portal venous phase scan taken only 40 seconds later than the scan in Fig. 5.12. The hypervascular lesion is no longer evident.

clearly demonstrates a hypervascular lesion within the liver, which is no longer evident on the portal venous phase scan (Fig. 5.13).

Imaging protocols vary, but, for optimal arterial enhancement, threshold-triggered scanning (around 30 seconds after injection), followed by a further acquisition around 65 seconds in the portal venous phase, is often advocated.

Parenchymal attenuation

A number of conditions can either increase (e.g. haemochromatosis) or decrease (e.g. fat infiltration) parenchymal attenuation. The attenuation of the unenhanced liver should be similar to that of the spleen. The liver is of decreased attenuation if the hepatic vessels are discernible from the background unenhanced liver.

Liver contour

The liver should have a smooth outline. A gross nodular outline may indicate tumour or macronodular cirrhosis, whereas a fine irregular outline may be associated with micronodular cirrhosis.

Biliary dilatation

The intrahepatic ducts are just discernible centrally. Generalized intrahepatic bile duct dilatation is typically caused by an obstruction of the extrahepatic bile duct system.

Focal lesions

The identification of focal lesions within the liver can be difficult. Precise diagnosis relies on the identification of morphological and enhancement characteristics, sometimes with the aid of other imaging modalities such as MRI and ultrasound. However, diffuse, infiltrating or very small lesions can be difficult to visualize against background liver. Other associated features must be actively sought. These features are summarized by system, below: biliary system, arterialization and portal veins.

Biliary system

Localized intrahepatic biliary dilatation may be due to compression by an underlying mass.

Look carefully for any evidence of biliary tract calculi or filling defects within the ducts. Check for the presence and appearance of the gallbladder. Look for air in the biliary tree – always an abnormal finding.

Arterialization

With continued growth of a focal mass, the lower-pressure portal veins are preferentially compressed and may become occluded. In this situation a distal wedge of liver acquires a preferential 'arterialized' supply. This is usually seen best in the late arterial phase, but sometimes persists into the portal venous phase. Attention should be paid to the lesion apex, where there may be a small tumour.

Conditions resulting in chronic compression of the liver parenchyma, such as an overlying rib, diaphragmatic fold or tense pericapsular fluid, may also result in arterialization.

Portal veins

Abrupt truncation of a portal vein branch can indicate a focal lesion.

Vessels

Assess the portal veins for evidence of truncation and thrombosis. Occasionally a splanchnic vessel aneurysm may be appreciated. Anomalies of hepatic arterial supply aid the surgeon in surgical planning or the radiologist in hepatic angiography.

Portal hypertension

The signs of portal hypertension include:

❏ venous collaterals and portosystemic varices – seen around the lower oesophagus, lesser gastric curve, rectal, lienorenal, falciform ligament and anterior abdominal wall
❏ portal vein enlargement (>16 mm) and thrombosis (Fig. 5.14)
❏ ascites
❏ splenomegaly.

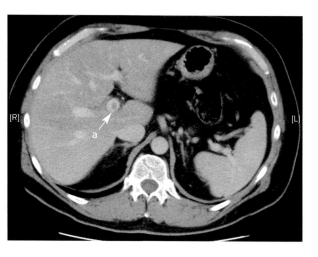

Fig. 5.14. Always follow the portal vein and its branches to the periphery. Note the low-attenuation thrombus within the contrast-opacified main portal vein (a).

Interpretation Tips

CT of the liver

● Perfusional changes. Areas of low attenuation on contrast-enhanced CT are often seen around the anterior aspect of the falciform ligament and gallbladder fossa. These areas are preferentially supplied by systemic veins and therefore fail to enhance on portal venous phase imaging. For the same reason, these areas are often the site of focal fatty sparing in the context of generalized liver fat infiltration.
● Focal fatty change is revealed as areas of decreased attenuation causing no distortion of underlying parenchyma with a predilection for the caudate lobe and perihilar areas. Distortion of the capsule and veins may imply a more sinister pathology and may require MRI to aid in diagnosis.
● The areas in the liver where pathology is often missed include: the left lobe underneath the left hemidiaphragm; the pericaval liver; and the caudate lobe.

> **QUICK REFERENCE CHECKLIST**
>
> ### CT of the liver and biliary tree
>
> Liver perfusion
> ● Phase of image acquisition and technical adequacy
> Parenchymal attenuation
> Liver contour
> Biliary dilatation
> Focal lesions
> ● Biliary system (calcified or non-calcified filling defects)
> ● Liver arterialization
> ● Truncation of portal veins
> Vessels
> ● Portal hypertension

UPPER ABDOMINAL ULTRASOUND

The following examination system is based on appraising organs sequentially, starting in the midline, moving across to the right upper quadrant and flank, and finishing at the left hypochondrium and flank. It is essential to give the patient clear instructions with regard to their breathing. Scan all organs in at least two planes and be able to adjust scanning parameters to optimize image quality.

Free fluid

Note whether free fluid is present within the upper abdomen.

Aorta

An aorta of less than 25 mm in diameter is considered normal, 25–30 mm ectatic and over 30 mm aneurysmal. If aortic dilatation is seen record:

❏ diameter – AP and transverse
❏ length and extent of dilatation – whether the iliac vessels are involved and whether supra- or infrarenal
❏ shape – fusiform or saccular
❏ presence of intramural thrombus.

Finally, look for para-aortic lymphadenopathy. If seen, search for further systemic lymphadenopathy and hepatosplenomegaly.

IVC

Note any obvious density within the IVC to suggest thrombus or tumour invasion. Dilatation (over 25 mm diameter) indicates right-heart failure. Also look for associated distension of the hepatic veins.

Pancreas

The pancreas is best viewed in transverse or transverse oblique section. The gland may not be seen well, owing to overlying gas. Therefore always record the adequacy of pancreatic visualization.

Evaluate:

❏ *reflectivity* – increases with age and may be heterogeneous due to calcification in chronic pancreatitis (CP)
❏ *outline* – irregular in CP
❏ *pancreatic duct* – if larger than 2 mm this indicates obstruction; ductal irregularity may be seen in CP
❏ *focal lesions* – carcinoma gives rise to low/mixed reflectivity lesions; anechoic pseudocysts may be seen in CP.

Liver

First look at the left, then the right lobe, using a combination of sagittal, transverse, subcostal and intercostal views.

Focal lesions

Systematically scan the liver for focal lesions. Below is a summary of the key ultrasound appearances of some of the more commonly encountered liver lesions.

Cysts
These may be single or multiple, with scalloped margins; they are well defined, anechoic and demonstrate posterior acoustic enhancement.

Haemangiomas
These are often small; they are well defined, highly reflective, classically peripheral and close to a vessel.

Metastases
Metastases are of variable appearance. They often have a surrounding halo of low reflectivity and ill-defined margins. They may displace and distort surrounding vessels (Fig. 5.15). They may display central necrosis. If metastases are suspected, this should prompt a search of the rest of the abdomen for a potential cause.

Hepatocellular carcinoma
This is of variable appearance on ultrasound, but there is invariably background liver disease. It frequently displays increased blood flow.

Focal fatty change
Focal fatty change is either fatty sparing within a fatty liver or focal fatty infiltration within a normal liver. Both are commonly found in segment 4, and cause no distortion of surrounding tissues.

Fig. 5.15. Typical rounded reflective 'target' metastases (a) within the liver secondary to a colonic primary carcinoma, adjacent to the gallbladder (b). Note the surrounding rim of low reflectivity.

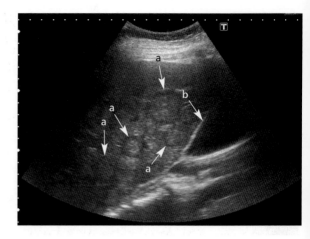

Abscesses

Abscesses are of variable appearance, depending on the stage of development. Later stages have an anechoic centre secondary to liquefaction.

Diffuse hepatic abnormality

After checking for focal lesions, decide whether there is a diffuse hepatic abnormality. Examples include:

❏ diffuse metastatic infiltration (Fig. 5.16)
❏ diffuse fatty infiltration
❏ cirrhosis (Fig. 5.17).

Diffuse fatty infiltration is common. It is characterized by generalized increased reflectivity and less well-defined portal tracts; deep liver detail is reduced owing to the attenuating properties of fat. Compare with renal parenchyma, which should be approximately isoechoic or marginally hypoechoic in relation to hepatic parenchyma.

Fig. 5.16. Here there is no normal liver parenchyma and therefore the diffuse abnormality can be missed. There is mixed, inhomogeneous, hepatic parenchymal echotexture secondary to widespread metastatic infiltration (a). Incidental note is made of gallstones (b) within the gallbladder, casting a dense acoustic shadow (c).

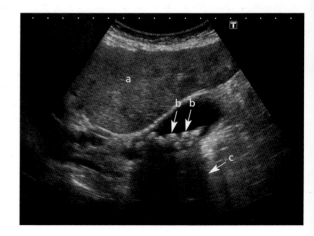

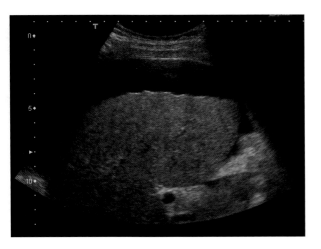

Fig. 5.17. Cirrhosis: ascites, coarse hepatic echotexture and an irregular capsular margin.

Potential changes seen in cirrhosis include:

❏ coarsened, reflective echotexture
❏ irregular capsular outline
❏ enlargement or reduction in size of the liver
❏ ascites
❏ portal hypertension, with reduced (<10 cm/s) or reversed portal vein flow, thrombus, coexistent varices and splenomegaly.

Gallbladder and biliary tree

Look for the following:

❏ *Biliary obstruction*. Are the intrahepatic ducts dilated? (Look for the 'double-barrel shotgun' sign of dilated bile ducts and accompanying portal vein.). Measure the extra-hepatic bile duct diameter (which is normally less than 7 mm pre-cholecystectomy, and 9 mm post-cholecystectomy). Obstruction should prompt the search for the cause (e.g. intraductal calculus, pancreatic head tumour or nodal enlargement). Fig. 5.18 demonstrates biliary obstruction secondary to a gallstone.
❏ *Gallbladder calculi*. These are highly mobile and reflective, and cast an acoustic shadow. A small, contracted gallbladder may be full of calculi, casting a dense acoustic shadow, and be difficult to discern from a gas-filled bowel loop.
❏ *Polyps*. These are of soft-tissue reflectivity and fixed to the wall without acoustic shadowing. Larger polyps (>10 mm) should be followed up by interval scanning, as they have pre-malignant potential. Look for localized wall thickening or a soft-tissue mass indicating potential cholangiocarcinoma.
❏ *Cholecystitis*. This is indicated by wall thickening (>3 mm when distended), layering and surrounding peri-cholecystic fluid. Calculi invariably accompany cholecystitis (Fig. 5.19). Gas within the gallbladder and gallbladder wall indicates emphysematous cholecystitis.

Fig. 5.18. Dilated common bile duct (a) secondary to an obstructing calculus (arrowed). Liver (b), pancreas (c). Note the dilated intrahepatic bile duct with its accompanying portal vein branch, the 'double-barrel shotgun' sign (d).

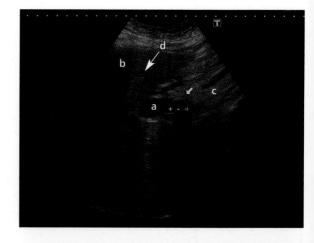

Fig. 5.19. Layered, thick-walled gallbladder (a) typical of acute cholecystitis. Note the rounded, echogenic calculus (b) with acoustic shadowing (c).

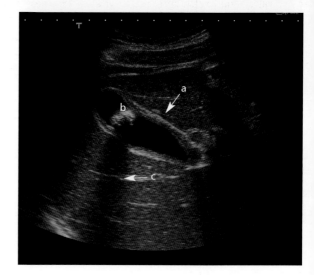

Kidneys

This is detailed separately in the next section 'Renal tract ultrasound', below (pp. 89–93).

Spleen

Assess size (normal is less than 12 cm). Causes of splenomegaly include portal hypertension, viral infections and systemic haematological conditions. If identified, search for a potential cause, such as signs of portal hypertension or lymphadenopathy.

Clues as to the aetiology of focal splenic lesions are given by their reflectivity:

❑ cysts are anechoic
❑ low-reflectivity lesions include infarcts, lymphomatous infiltration and haematomas
❑ high-reflectivity lesions include haemangiomas, post-infection scarring or calcification following tuberculosis
❑ splenic metastases show variable, mixed reflectivity.

Interpretation Tips

Upper abdominal ultrasound

● If pathology is identified, look hard for associated features – do not be satisfied with one positive finding alone. For example, in cirrhosis, look for all the signs of portal hypertension. If lymphadenopathy is identified, look for a potential cause.
● Move the patient from supine to the left lateral position to differentiate polyps from calculi and to dislodge calculi hidden within the neck of the gallbladder.
● Gastrointestinal metastases tend to give rise to hyperechoic liver lesions.

QUICK REFERENCE CHECKLIST

Upper abdominal ultrasound

Free fluid
Aorta
IVC
Pancreas
● Reflectivity
● Outline
● Pancreatic duct
● Focal lesions
Liver
● Focal lesions
● Diffuse hepatic abnormality
Gallbladder and biliary tree
● Biliary obstruction
● Calculi
● Polyps
● Cholecystitis
Kidneys
Spleen

RENAL TRACT ULTRASOUND

Indications for renal tract scanning include renal failure, obstruction, haematuria, masses, loin pain and calculus disease.

The kidneys should always be scanned in both longitudinal and transverse planes. The right kidney is often easier to visualize than the left, and a combination of moving both the patient and the probe, and getting the patient to hold their breath, is often required to see both kidneys clearly.

Renal size

Measure renal length. The normal kidney measures 9–12 cm, dependent on age and build. The left kidney is often 0.5–1 cm larger than the right.

Renal outline

The renal outline should be smooth. Both normal variants (e.g. splenic hump and persistent fetal lobulation) and pathology (e.g. scars and infarcts) can lead to an irregular renal outline.

Renal parenchymal thickness

The renal parenchyma consists of the renal cortex and medullary pyramids. The distance between the capsule and the high-reflectivity renal sinus fat decreases with age and chronic renal disease. It is generally accepted that a thickness of less than 1.3 cm is abnormal.

Renal cortical reflectivity

The renal cortex is normally isoechoic or hypoechoic in comparison with the liver. Increased parenchymal reflectivity indicates nephritis; however, this is a non-specific finding (Fig. 5.20).

Fig. 5.20. Increased renal cortical reflectivity indicating nephritis. Note how the renal cortex (a) is more reflective than the hepatic parenchyma (b), and consequently the low-reflectivity medullary pyramids (c) appear more prominent.

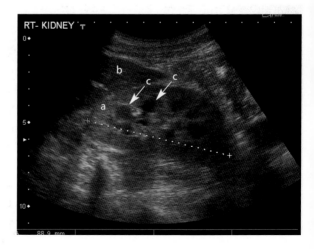

Renal masses

Search for mass lesions. Small renal cell carcinomas can be hard to detect as they are often isoechoic to the surrounding parenchyma. Larger renal cell carcinomas become more heterogeneous and distort the renal outline.

A well-defined area displaying markedly increased reflectivity is likely to represent an angiomyolipoma.

Benign simple cysts are very common with increasing age. Look for septations or surrounding thickening and irregularity, which may represent the solid component of a cystic renal cell carcinoma.

Renal calcification

Try to discern renal parenchymal calcification from calculi within the collecting system. As the surrounding renal sinus is highly reflective, small calculi can be hard to detect. Look for highly reflective, rounded foci casting an acoustic shadow (Fig. 5.21). Arcuate vessels, which can be highly reflective and have a characteristic 'double echo' representing both walls of the vessel, should not be confused with calculi.

Collecting system

Look for pelvi-calyceal dilatation (Fig. 5.22). Beware that this may be physiological (e.g. overfull bladder, pregnancy or prominent extrarenal pelvis) as well as pathological (obstruction and reflux). Clinical acumen will help to elucidate a cause. For example, if bilateral pelvicalyceal dilatation is seen in a male patient, this should prompt the search for an enlarged prostate, as it may obstruct bladder outflow.

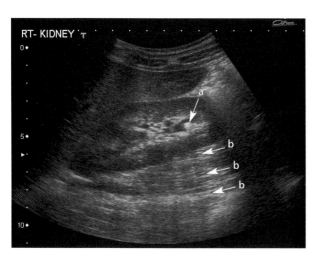

Fig. 5.21. Rounded, reflective calculus (a) within a dilated lower pole calyx in the right kidney. Although not easy to spot, the acoustic shadowing (b) confirms the diagnosis.

Fig. 5.22. Hydronephrosis of the right kidney demonstrating a dilated calyx (a), pelvis (b) and upper ureter (c).

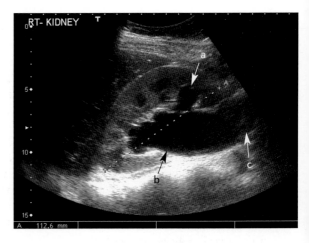

Renal vascularity

Assessing renal vascularity using Doppler is technically difficult and notoriously unreliable in inexperienced hands. Renal artery stenosis is indicated by increased flow velocity at the site of occlusion, with a slow arterial upstroke on the spectral analysis distal to the stenosis.

If venous thrombosis is suspected, look for clot within the dilated renal vein; colour Doppler may demonstrate reduced or absent flow. The spectral trace typically shows absent or reversed flow in diastole.

Perirenal area

Do not forget to search for adrenal masses and perirenal lesions.

Pre-micturition bladder

Scan in both the sagittal and transverse planes. Search for debris, clot and calculi. Note the wall thickness (normally under 3 mm if well distended), and specifically note any localized wall thickening suggestive of transitional cell carcinoma. If obstruction is suspected, use colour Doppler to identify ureteric jets. Search for surrounding free fluid.

Post-micturition bladder

The assessment of residual volume is particularly important in the presence of suspected prostatic hypertrophy or neurogenic bladder dysfunction. Calculate by multiplying the product of the width, length and transverse diameter by 0.52. Over 50 ml is considered abnormal.

Interpretation Tips

Renal tract ultrasound

- If views are difficult, move the patient into oblique and lateral positions.
- The renal hilum and pelvicalyceal system are best viewed in the coronal plane.
- Using a higher-frequency probe with thin patients can accentuate acoustic shadowing by small, equivocal calculi.
- Do not forget to use colour Doppler on mass lesions to demonstrate vascularity.
- Moving the patient into a lateral position will confirm whether a bladder lesion is mobile (e.g. calculus) or fixed (e.g. transitional cell carcinoma).
- If a suspected renal cell carcinoma is identified, examine the contralateral kidney carefully, as synchronous tumours are common.

QUICK REFERENCE CHECKLIST

Renal tract ultrasound

Renal size
Renal outline
Renal parenchymal thickness
Renal cortical reflectivity
Renal masses
Renal calcification
Collecting system
Renal vascularity
Perirenal area
Pre-micturition bladder
Post-micturition bladder

TRANSABDOMINAL ULTRASOUND OF THE FEMALE PELVIS

Indications for this commonly requested investigation include pelvic and lower abdominal pain, vaginal bleeding and palpable pelvic masses. To a certain extent, focused gynaecological ultrasound (specifically transvaginal ultrasound) is becoming the preserve of the specialist radiologist, sonographer or gynaecologist. It none the less still remains important for those performing general ultrasound on a day-to-day basis to recognize common gynaecological and lower abdominal pathology.

A full bladder is essential for transabdominal scanning, as it provides an acoustic window through which to view the pelvic organs. It is helpful to note the stage of the menstrual cycle, as this will influence interpretation.

Uterus

View the uterus in both transverse and longitudinal sections. Assess:

❏ size (overall length and width of the body)
❏ endometrial thickness at the fundus
❏ congenital uterine abnormalities such as a septate or bicornuate uterus
❏ the presence of an intrauterine contraceptive device
❏ uterine position (i.e. anteverted or retroverted).

Look specifically for endometrial and myometrial pathology.

Endometrium

Identify focal endometrial thickening. Premenopausal endometrial thickness should be less than 14 mm, dependent on the stage of the menstrual cycle. With post-menopausal bleeding, an endometrial thickening over 4 mm, in the absence of hormone replacement therapy, raises the possibility of malignancy.

A diffusely thickened endometrium containing cystic areas is typical of endometrial hyperplasia.

Look for polyps projecting into the endometruim.

Myometrium

Fibroids (leiomyomata) are common. They display a well-defined, spherical or lobulated outline and may have a low-reflectivity centre indicating central necrosis. Calcification within fibroids is common. Note whether fibroids are subserosal (project outwards), contained within the myometrium, submucosal (project into the endometrial cavity) or situated within the cervix. Malignant transformation into leiomyosarcoma is very rare.

Asymmetrical myometrial thickening with cystic areas in the absence of a discernible mass lesion is typical of adenomyosis.

Ovaries

Because of their variable position within the pelvis, the ovaries can be difficult to locate on transabdominal scanning. Start scanning in the transverse plane above the symphysis, angling down into the pelvis. Then tilt the probe upwards to locate the ovaries, which are often adjacent to the filled bladder. Assess ovarian size and identify any cysts or mass lesions.

Size

Normal ovarian volumes are 6–12 ml in the reproductive age group and below 4 ml in postmenopausal women.

Simple cysts

Simple cysts in the reproductive age group are likely to represent physiological follicles and should be reported as such to avoid provoking anxiety. Normal dominant follicles measure approximately 8–25 mm in diameter before ovulation.

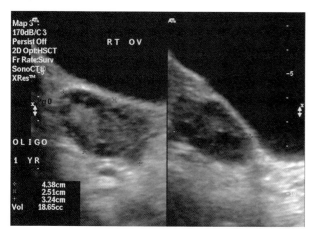

Fig. 5.23. Polycystic ovaries. Magnified transverse and sagittal views of the right ovary. The ovarian volume is increased (>12 ml) and there are multiple (>12), small (<1 cm), peripherally sited cysts.

Larger cysts within postmenopausal ovaries often require ultrasound follow-up to ensure that no change has occurred.

Large-volume ovaries with multiple (over 12) peripherally situated cysts less than 1 cm in size are termed 'polycystic' (Fig. 5.23).

Mass lesions

It is often difficult to definitively characterize an ovarian mass as benign or malignant. If a mass is identified, describe:

❏ its size, shape and outline
❏ whether it is predominantly solid or cystic or mixed
❏ the echotexture of solid elements
❏ its vascularity (from colour Doppler).

The presence of a predominantly cystic mass containing irregular solid elements with increased vascularity is typical of malignancy.

Some benign lesions have characteristic appearances such as dermoid tumours (solid mass displaying mixed-reflectivity areas of fat and calcification) and endometriomas (well-defined lesions displaying speckled, uniform, low reflectivity).

Fig. 5.24 demonstrates an ovarian adenocarcinoma.

Pouch of Douglas and adnexa

Note any free fluid within the dependent pelvic spaces. A low-reflectivity, complex mass may represent an abscess related to pelvic inflammatory disease. Endometriomas are commonly found within the pouch of Douglas and adnexa.

A fluid-filled tubular structure within the adnexal region may well represent an obstructed fallopian tube (hydrosalpinx).

Fig. 5.24. Large, predominantly cystic mass within the pelvis displaying septations (a), solid elements (b) and wall thickening inferiorly (c). Doppler imaging demonstrated blood flow within the solid elements. This lesion was subsequently confirmed to be ovarian adenocarcinoma.

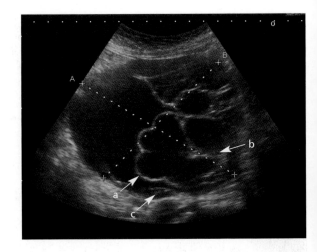

Bladder

Review the bladder for focal mural thickening, debris/calculi and dilatation of the distal ureters.

Bowel

Do not neglect to look for a bowel-related cause of lower abdominal pain. Right iliac fossa pain may be due to inflammatory bowel disease, malignancy or appendicitis. It is the author's experience that a common indication is the differential diagnosis of right iliac fossa pain in females, which is between appendicitis and right-sided tubal/ovarian pathology. In this circumstance, use compression and a high-frequency

Fig. 5.25. Consider other, non-gynaecological causes of lower abdominal pain. This ultrasound, performed with a high-frequency linear probe, shows the transverse view of an oedematous, inflamed appendix (a), surrounded by high-reflectivity fat with adjacent free fluid (b).

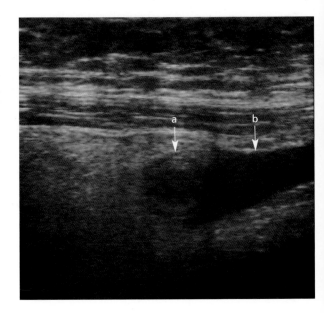

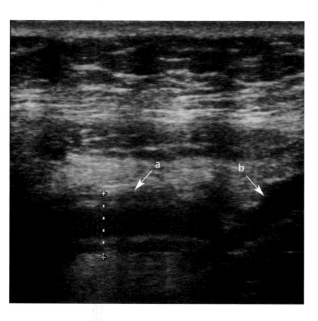

Fig. 5.26. The longitudinal view of the appendix (a) with adjacent free fluid (b) shown in Fig. 5.25.

linear probe to search for a thickened, blind-ending loop of non-compressible bowel to confirm an inflamed appendix (Figs 5.25 and 5.26).

Left iliac fossa pain can be due to tumour, diverticulitis or abscess. Although gas makes bowel visualization tricky, look hard for collections and bowel wall thickening (over 4 mm) with compression views.

Interpretation Tips

Transabdominal ultrasound of the female pelvis

- Mixed solid/cystic masses demonstrating vascularity strongly suggest malignancy.
- Unexpected pregnancy is a common cause of lower abdominal symptoms. A gestational sac should be visible 5 weeks after the end of the last period.
- Interval scanning of an ovarian cyst of uncertain aetiology, at a different stage of the menstrual cycle, can often resolve the diagnosis.
- Look for local invasion or distant spread (e.g. ascites or liver metastases) when a possible malignancy is identified.
- If a typical polycystic ovary is identified, this does not necessarily indicate polycystic ovarian syndrome (PCOS), and conversely it is possible to have morphologically normal ovaries in PCOS.

QUICK REFERENCE CHECKLIST

Transabdominal ultrasound of the female pelvis

Uterus
● Endometrium
● Myometrium
Ovaries
● Size
● Simple cysts
● Mass lesions
Pouch of Douglas and adnexa
Bladder
Bowel

SCROTAL ULTRASOUND

Scrotal ultrasound is performed with a high-frequency linear probe (7.5–10 MHz). Scan both testes and epididymides in longitudinal and transverse planes.

Scrotal wall

Briefly assess the thickness of the scrotal wall. Generalized thickening can occur in oedema due to heart failure. Localized thickening may be due to inflammation or infection.

Fig. 5.27. Fluid surrounding the testis; typical appearances of a simple hydrocele.

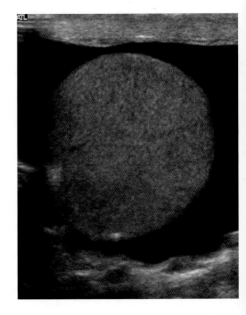

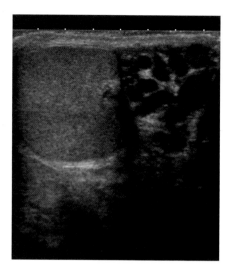

Fig. 5.28. Left-sided varicocele. Dilated testicular veins adjacent to the left testis.

Paratesticular fluid

A small amount of fluid around the testicle is normal. Fluid surrounding more than half the testicular circumference is a hydrocele (Fig. 5.27).

Varicocele

Look for dilatation of the veins of the spermatic cord. To confirm the diagnosis, use Doppler to demonstrate venous distension and increased flow on Valsalva manoeuvre (Fig. 5.28).

Epidydimal pathology

Evaluate the size, echotexture and vascularity of each epididymis.

Symmetrical epididymal tubular dilatation is a normal post-vasectomy finding.

Epididymitis

This is seen as a swollen epididymis (typically tail), of mixed reflectivity and increased vascularity with or without orchitis and reactive hydrocele. Previous inflammation may lead to epididymal calcification.

Cysts

These are common and either represent a spermatocele – dilatation of efferent ductules containing sperm and proteinaceous material predominantly in the epididymal head – or epididymal cysts (serous fluid).

Tumours

Tumours show mixed reflectivity and are mostly adenomas. Malignant tumours are extremely rare.

Testes

Evaluate the size, morphology, echotexture and vascularity of each testis. Decide whether there is a generalized or focal abnormality.

Generalized pathology

Orchitis
Features include swelling of the testis, patchy low reflectivity, accentuation of septal architecture and hypervascularity. Orchitis is invariably associated with epididymitis.

Torsion
Few grey-scale findings are seen in early torsion. The hallmark is reduced or absent blood flow on Doppler.

Trauma
Trauma produces mixed-reflectivity areas of haemorrhage and oedema. Look for rupture of the tunica albuginea. Use Doppler to evaluate the vascularity (viability) of the affected testis.

Testicular microlithiasis
More than five foci of calcification, of less than 2 mm, within each testis are considered abnormal. There is a putative association with testicular malignancy and annual follow-up is recommended in young men.

Focal pathology

Malignancy
Seminoma (generally rounded, hypoechoic, homogeneous and confined within the tunica at presentation) and teratoma (well defined, commonly with cystic elements

Fig. 5.29. Multifocal seminoma on a background of testicular microlithiasis. This longitudinal view of the testis shows several ill-defined, low-reflectivity lesions (a) and numerous small, high-reflectivity microcalcifications (b).

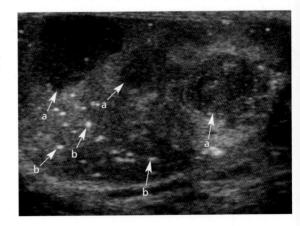

and calcification) are seen. Both distort underlying testicular architecture. Infrequently, lymphoma can present as low-reflectivity focal testicular lesions.

Fig. 5.29 demonstrates a multifocal neoplasm.

Benign lesions
Simple cysts appear as well-defined, thin-walled, anechoic areas with distal acoustic enhancement. Other benign lesions can present as focal testicular masses, such as adrenal rests and epidermoids, but these are rare.

Calcification
Causes of focal calcification include inflammation, malignancy and previous trauma.

Inguinal region

If suggested by the history, look in the inguinal region for an indirect inguinal hernia protruding into the scrotum.

Interpretation Tips

Scrotal ultrasound

● Ask the patient to locate small scrotal masses if you have failed to identify their position initially.
● Demonstrate both testicles in the same image for a direct comparison of parenchymal reflectivity.
● Rarely, left-sided varicocele is associated with renal malignancy (as the left testicular vein drains into the left renal vein); therefore left renal scanning is indicated.
● If a hydrocele is apparent, then search for an underlying cause (e.g. mass lesion or infection).
● Spontaneous de-torsion is recognized, so do not be falsely reassured by normal vascularity in the presence of a high clinical suspicion of testicular torsion.

QUICK REFERENCE CHECKLIST

Scrotal ultrasound

Scrotal wall
Paratesticular fluid
Varicocele
Epididymal pathology
Testes
• Generalized pathology
• Focal pathology
Inguinal region

MUSCULOSKELETAL RADIOLOGY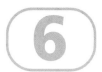

INTRODUCTION TO MUSCULOSKELETAL IMAGING
Fractures

Figs 6.1 and 6.2 provides an example of a severe injury.

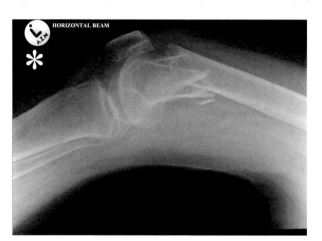

Fig. 6.1. Lateral view of a comminuted fracture of the distal left femoral diaphysis. There is intra-articular extension, medial displacement and posterior angulation. The bones are generally osteopenic.

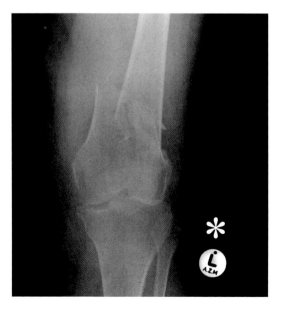

Fig. 6.2. Anteroposterior view of the comminuted fracture shown in Fig. 6.1.

Identification of the fracture

Radiological signs of a fracture include:

- ❏ lucent line – distraction of bone fragments
- ❏ sclerotic line – impaction of bone fragments
- ❏ trabecular disruption
- ❏ cortical buckling (torus fracture).

In children look for:

- ❏ bending of bone
- ❏ growth plate disruption (Salter–Harris fractures – see Chapter 8).

Site

Comment on the following:

- ❏ left or right
- ❏ bones involved
- ❏ site within bone – epiphysis (head), metaphysis (neck), diaphysis (shaft) (alternatively divide long bones into proximal, middle and distal thirds).

Bone quality

State whether the fracture is pathological as a result of metabolic, neoplastic or infectious disease.

Age of injury

State whether there is any evidence of healing in the form of bridging callus, or sclerosis of the bone ends, which implies an established non-union.

Number of fragments

A fracture that results in the production of two bone fragments is termed a 'simple fracture'. If more than two fragments result, then the fracture is described as comminuted, though in practice the term is reserved for fractures with innumerable fragments. It is also acceptable to describe three-part, four-part fractures and so on.

Articular involvement

Intra-articular fractures are more prone to arthritic change and often require surgical fixation to restore joint congruity than extra-articular fractures.

Fracture type

Describe the fracture pattern. Certain types of fracture are inherently more stable than others.

❏ *Hairline*. Undisplaced fractures following minimal trauma may be apparent by the presence of only fine cortical branching lucency, periosteal reaction or soft-tissue swelling. Stress fractures are generally of this type.

❏ *Greenstick*. These occur predominantly in children. They result in buckling of the bone on one side only.

❏ *Transverse*. This is a single fracture line running either perpendicularly to the long axis of the bone or with an obliquity <30°.

❏ *Spiral*. A spiral fracture line usually results from a torsion force and is often un-stable.

❏ *Oblique*. The fracture line is angled obliquely (>30°).

❏ *Avulsion*. This denotes a fragment of bone that has been 'pulled off' at the site of a ligament or tendon insertion.

❏ *Depression*. This denotes a depression of a fragment of a flat bone surface (e.g. skull, tibial plateau).

❏ *Impaction*. This describes a decrease in the width or height of a bone due to fragments being driven into each other. Impaction is most often due to axial loading, for example on the vertebra or calcaneus.

Deformity

Describing deformity is important, as this influences management. The degree of deformity correlates with neurovascular injury. Deformity is described with respect to the standard anatomical position and, unless specified, relates to the position of the distal fragment.

Displacement (i.e. the presence of translational deformity)

Displacement can also be quantified by the approximate percentage of bone apposition (e.g. 0% bone apposition, implying an 'off-ended' fracture). The terms 'anterior', 'posterior', 'lateral' and 'medial' are used to describe the direction of displacement. There are some special cases, however:

❏ *The forearm and hand*. The terms 'volar' and 'dorsal' are used instead of anterior and posterior. Radial and ulnar are used in place of lateral and medial, respectively.

❏ *Shortening*. Shortening is a type of displacement in which the presence of overriding, overlapping fragments results in shortening of the affected bone or limb.

❏ *Axial rotation*. This is often difficult to determine radiologically but is more obvious when the joints above and below are visualized.

Angulation

Angulation of a fracture is used to describe the orientation of the distal fragment. Both the direction and amount of angulation (the angle with respect to the normal long bone axis) should be described.

As before, the terms 'volar', 'dorsal', 'radial' and 'ulnar' are generally used in the hand and forearm.

Additionally in the lower limb the outward and inward angulation of the distal part of the limb are termed 'valgus' and 'varus angulation', respectively.

Soft tissue

The presence of soft-tissue swelling may indicate a radiologically occult underlying fracture. The presence of soft-tissue disruption could indicate a compound (open) fracture.

Interpretation Tips

Fractures

● A fracture may not be discernible on a single view. Always compare at least two views.
● Accessory ossicles can occasionally be confused for avulsion fractures. Clinical correlation is important. Ossicles are smooth and corticated whereas avulsion fragments are not corticated on all sides. It is important to become familiar with common sites of accessory ossicles.
● Impacted fractures are sometimes only visible as an area of sclerosis

---

QUICK REFERENCE CHECKLIST

Fractures

Site
Bone quality
Age of injury
Number of fragments
Articular involvement
Fracture type
Deformity
● Displacement
● Angulation
Soft tissue

Radiological characterization of bone lesions

When faced with a bone lesion, a systematic appraisal of the radiological features can considerably narrow the differential diagnosis:

❑ patient age – certain lesions are more common in children and others more common in adults

❏ whether the lesion is solitary or multiple
❏ whether the lesion is predominantly sclerotic or lytic
❏ the site of the lesion – whether the lesion is epiphyseal, metaphyseal or diaphy-
   seal, and whether it is based in medullary or cortical bone, or the periosteum.

Some lesions have a predilection for a particular bone.

Table 6.1 sets out some criteria by which to judge whether a lesion is benign or
aggressive. ('Aggressive' is used here in place of 'malignant' because not all such
lesions are neoplastic. The term 'aggressive' merely implies rapidity of progres-
sion.)

Table 6.1. Radiological characteristics of benign and aggressive lesions

	Benign	Aggressive
Margin	Well defined, with or without a sclerotic rim	Ill defined, permeative
Cortical involvement	None – lesion grows along medulla and thus may appear ovoid. Typical of slow-growing lesions	Endosteal scalloping (i.e. erosion of the inner side of the cortex)
	Cortical expansion – thinning of the endosteal cortex and laying down of new periosteal bone is almost always due to slow-growing, uniform, expansile lesions, which may give the impression of an expanded cortex	Cortical breach
Periosteal reaction	Smooth, well defined. May be single or multilayered	Various types causing reactive, ill-defined formation of new bone
Zone of transition	Well-defined, narrow zone of transition between normal and abnormal bone	Wide zone of transition, ill defined and permeative
Matrix calcification (mineralization of the underlying tumour matrix)	Occasionally seen	Generally absent

Figs 6.3 and 6.4 demonstrate examples of benign and malignant lesions, respectively.

Interpretation Tip

Characterization of bone lesions

● None of the above features is absolutely diagnostic, but the combination of features
  should point the reporting radiologist in a particular direction.

Fig. 6.3. Features of a benign lesion – fibrous dysplasia. There is cortical expansion of this predominantly lytic lesion. It is well defined, with a narrow zone of transition; the cortex is intact, and there is no associated periosteal reaction.

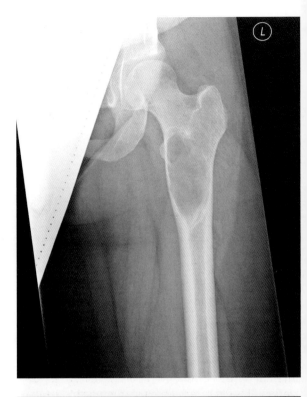

Fig. 6.4. Features of an aggressive lesion – osteosarcoma. Note ill-defined sclerosis in the proximal tibial metaphysis and diaphysis, cortical breach, marked periosteal reaction and a wide zone of transition distally.

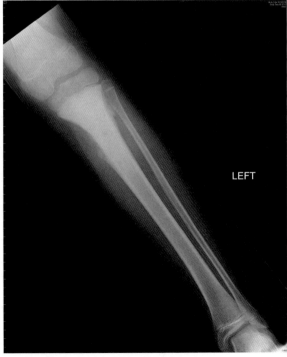

QUICK REFERENCE CHECKLIST

Characterization of bone lesions

Patient age
Solitary or multiple
Predominant density
Site
Benign or aggressive features
● Margin
● Cortical involvement
● Periosteal border
● Zone of transition
● Matrix calcification

Postoperative radiography

Types of fracture fixation

Internal fixation
Internal fixation is used for fractures that require accurate reduction or early mobilization. It is important for the radiologist to have a basic working knowledge of fixation devices and the complications associated with their use.

❏ *Screws/pins*. Simple screw fixation is used for the reattachment of small bone fragments, such as in the malleoli.
❏ *Dynamic hip screw*. A special type of screw used for intratrochanteric fractures of the femoral neck that allows dynamic fracture compression and potential rapid healing.
❏ *Plate fixation*. This is often used in combination with screws to enable a stronger fixation, often resulting in good compression across the fracture.
❏ *Intramedullary nailing*. Nailing through the medullary cavity of a long bone, across the fracture site, enables good fixation and early mobilization.
❏ *Wires*. These are used in the reduction of small bones.
❏ *Stiff Kirschner (K) wires*. These are used in the distal forearm, the hand and the foot.
❏ *Encircling tension band wires*. These are used to provide fracture compression where the natural range of motion produces a distracting force across the fracture (e.g. in the olecranon and patella).

External fixation
External fixation is often used for fractures with associated soft-tissue and vascular injury or contaminated wounds. It is indicated to avoid further damage to an already compromised limb or to minimize the risk of prosthetic infection.

Arthroplasty

Arthroplasty techniques are continually evolving and there is considerable variation in the appearance and placement of different prostheses. Be guided by the clinical history and any technical information from the operating surgeon.

Type of prosthesis

Try to identify the type of prosthesis. Any prosthesis may be a combination of the types listed below. A joint may be replaced with a variety of materials, including metal alloys, polymers and ceramics.

Total joint replacement, hemiarthroplasty and bipolar hemiarthroplasty   A joint replacement is defined as total if both articular surfaces are replaced.

A hemiarthroplasty involves replacement of one articular surface.

Bipolar hemiarthroplasty, commonly used in hip replacements, is a single component that permits motion between the metal head and inner polyethylene socket, as well as the outer metallic cup and the acetabulum.

Unicompartmental arthroplasty   If degenerative joint disease preferentially affects one side of the joint, then a unicompartmental arthroplasty can be used to replace both articular surfaces on this side. The technique is most commonly used in unicompartmental (either medial or lateral) disease of the knee.

Resurfacing arthroplasty   Resurfacing arthroplasty aims simply to resurface the arthritic surface of a joint. This involves less bone removal than a total replacement and is generally used in younger patients, who may require subsequent revision.

Revision arthroplasty   Revision arthroplasty is occasionally indicated if the original components are worn or infected. These have a wide range of appearances but usually involve the use of larger, more substantial prostheses.

Cement   Comment on the presence or absence of cement. Non-cemented implants are designed to allow bone in-growth and to reduce the incidence of loosening.

Postoperative complications

Radiology plays an important role in the identification of complications from joint replacements, so assess every prosthesis for evidence of complications. It is beyond the scope of this book to outline the appearances of all device complications and the general principles follow.

Previous imaging

Seek out previous images. Complications often evolve slowly and serial images taken over time can considerably aid interpretation.

Early complications
On an immediate postoperative image look for malposition, intraoperative fracture and cement extrusion.

Malposition   The criteria for satisfactory surgical placement vary with the device used.

❏ *Stem position*. Any stem should generally pass straight down the longitudinal bone axis. Any abnormality of position here predisposes to periprosthetic fracture and loosening.
❏ *Cup position*. Abnormalities in the positioning of a prosthetic cup (e.g. the acetabulum) limit the range of motion and predispose to dislocation.

Intraoperative fracture   Fractures occur in 2–10% of cases. These are often of the subtle, hairline type.

Cement extrusion   This is usually asymptomatic but can cause thermal injury to soft tissues.

Late complications
The value of previous images here cannot be overemphasized. Painful arthroplasties may be due to a number of problems, including loosening, dislocation, infection, component failure and osseous abnormality.

Loosening   Loosening results from abnormalities in the binding at the prosthesis–cement–bone interface. Look for:

❏ increasing lucency over sequential radiographs
❏ wide focal lucency at interfaces (a lucent zone <2 mm parallel to the bone margin is acceptable)
❏ cement fragmentation
❏ migration or sinking of the prosthesis (this is diagnostic of loosening but detection of subtle migration often requires comparison with a baseline image)
❏ endosteal scalloping or periosteal reaction at the tip or stem of the prosthesis.

Dislocation   Factors predisposing to dislocation include malposition of the components and abnormalities of the musculature.

Periprosthetic fracture   Periprosthetic fracture often occurs around the stem or distal tip of a prosthesis, and can be of the stress or insufficiency type.

Heterotopic ossification   This is an exuberant ossification in the soft tissue, which can occur after trauma or surgery. The mechanisms are poorly understood.

Infection   Radiographically, infection resembles loosening, with progressive bone lysis. Occasionally gas in the soft tissue may be seen.

Fig. 6.5 is an image of a chronically painful right hip due to an infected joint replacement.

Fig. 6.5. Chronically infected right total hip replacement. There is lucency surrounding the stem of the prosthesis (a) and associated sclerosis and periosteal reaction (b).

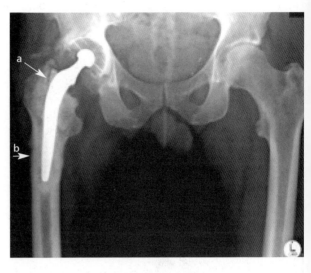

Component failure   Components occasionally fracture.

QUICK REFERENCE CHECKLIST

Postoperative complications

Previous imaging
Early complications
● Malposition
● Intraoperative fracture
● Cement extrusion
Late complications
● Loosening
● Dislocation
● Periprosthetic fracture
● Heterotopic ossification
● Infection
● Component failure

JOINT RADIOLOGY

Conventionally, arthritis has been viewed as a primary disease of cartilage, but increasingly it has been recognized that cartilage change is secondary to either synovial or bone marrow changes.

The diagnosis of joint disease is essentially a multidisciplinary one and relies on clinical, radiological, biochemical and pathological correlation.

Fig. 6.6 shows the radiographic features of chronic joint disease.

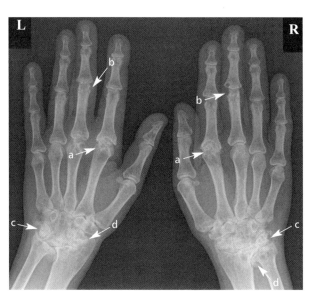

Fig. 6.6. Radiograph of the hand, demonstrating erosive rheumatoid arthritis with secondary degenerative changes. Symmetrical small joint polyarthritis. Note periarticular erosions at the metacarphalangeal joints (a) and proximal interphalangeal joints (b), with associated loss of joint space and soft-tissue swelling, collapse of the proximal carpal row (c), and secondary degenerative changes, including at the radiocarpal and distal radioulnar joints (d).

Patient age and sex

Diseases may occur with greater frequency in children, or younger or older adults. Certain diseases display a sex predilection.

Disease distribution

Note whether:

❏ the disease distribution is symmetrical or non-symmetrical
❏ the axial skeleton and/or the sacroiliac joints are affected
❏ predominantly small or large joints are affected
❏ there is single-joint (monoarthropathy) or multiple-joint (polyarthropathy) involvement.

Joint space narrowing

Narrowing of the joint space is indicative of cartilage destruction and is seen in a number of the arthritides. Note the distribution of the narrowing and whether it affects a particular joint compartment. In the early stages of osteoarthritis, the narrowing is confined to the load-bearing areas of the joint.

Articular bone

Changes in the underlying bone can be broadly divided into atrophic (bone lysis) and bone forming.

Atrophic (bone lysis) changes

Osteoporosis   Decide whether the demineralization is global or periarticular.

Erosions   The location of erosions can give a clue as to the aetiology:

❏ *Marginal*. At the point of capsular insertions, in the 'bare area' of the bone within the synovial space not covered by cartilage. This implies a synovial origin.
❏ *Articular*. Erosions of the articular surface are seen at points of focally increased pressure.
❏ *Juxta-articular*. Erosions are located away from the joint.
❏ *Distant*. Erosions at the points of tendinous insertion are sometimes seen in tenosynovitis.

Subchondral cysts   Well-circumscribed defects in the subarticular bone are seen in a variety of joint disorders.

Bone-forming changes

Bone-forming changes can be classified as either 'buttressing' changes, which increase the stability of the joint but at the expense range of movement, or 'interface' changes (reactive changes at the overlap region of the periosteum, joint capsule and bone).

Buttressing changes   Buttressing changes include:

❏ subchondral sclerosis – reactive new bone formation just deep to the cartilage layer
❏ the appearance of osteophytes.

Interface changes   Syndesmophytes are calcifications of the outer fibres of the intervertebral discs resulting in paravertebral bony ossification that runs vertically, as opposed to osteophytes, which run horizontally. They can be classified as symmetrical/non-symmetrical (best seen on the AP projection) and marginal/non-marginal. Marginal syndesmophytes originate from the edge of a vertebral end-plate. Non-marginal syndesmophytes originate from the vertebral body away from the end-plate.

Periosteal reactions are seen in fewer than 2% of cases of rheumatoid arthritis and 5–10% of cases of psoriatic arthritis. They are also seen in tumours, infection and post-traumatic conditions.

In addition, chondrocalcinosis (calcification of the joint cartilage) can lead to secondary degenerative joint disease and is seen in the crystal deposition syndromes.

Interpretation Tips

Joints

● In any radiograph of the leg, note whether it was taken while the patient was weight bearing, as this affects the width of the joint space.

● Although some images will display 'classic' features of a specific form of arthritis, considerable overlap exists and it is often frustrating and futile to try to shoehorn a 'non-classic' constellation of findings. Fig. 6.7 illustrates the degree of overlap between the arthritides.

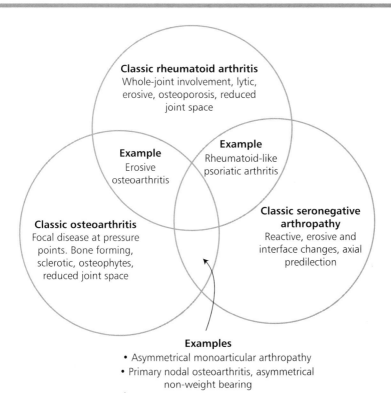

Fig. 6.7. The overlap in the radiographic appearance of the arthritides.

Disease complications

Progressive disease can result in joint deformity, often secondary to cartilage destruction or tendon or ligament instability. There are several types.

❑ *Angulation*. If there is asymmetrical loading through a joint, the resulting osteoarthritis can lead to angulation of the affected joint or limb.

❏ *Ankylosis*. This is joint stiffness secondary to osseous or fibrous bridging in end-stage arthritis.
❏ *Malalignment*. Inflammatory arthropathy can result in ligament and tendon laxity, leading to subluxation, dislocation and deformity.
❏ *Bone resorption*. Severe erosive arthropathy with extensive bone resorption can result in soft-tissue collapse.

Soft tissue

Swelling
Symmetrical fusiform swelling seen on plain film is indicative of active inflammation and arthritis.

Effusion
Displaced tissue and fat planes may suggest a joint effusion, but in reality this is a poor discriminator of disease.

APPENDICULAR RADIOGRAPHY

General approach to the appendicular plain radiograph

The general points of interpretation outlined below can be applied to all appendicular plain films, and for the purpose of brevity will not be repeated for each extremity body part. The order of review may vary depending on the image; however, the principles of interpretation remain the same. It pays to become familiar with the appearances of normal variants and to have ready reference to an appropriate atlas.

Adequacy

Is the area of concern adequately covered? Do the joints above and below need to be seen and are there two views? Ascertain whether the images are true AP, oblique or lateral, as the correct projection can be critical for successful interpretation.

Overview

An initial review will detect gross pathology, such as displaced fractures, dislocations and conspicuous bone tumours. Make an overall assessment of the alignment and the quality of the bone. For example, is the bone mineralization normal? Note previous metalwork after internal fixation (see 'Postoperative radiography – postoperative complications', pp. 110–112). The finding of an abnormality on the initial overview should not preclude a thorough systematic search for associated or additional subtle pathology.

Alignment

Check bone alignment. More detailed assessment of alignment relating to individual components of the appendicular skeleton is covered in the following pages.

Joints

Patient age and sex
Disease distribution
Articular bone
Joint space narrowing
● Atrophic (bone lysis) changes
 – Osteoporosis
 – Erosions
 – Subchondral cysts
● Bone-forming changes
 – Buttressing change (subchondral sclerosis, osteophytes)
 – Interface changes (syndesmophytes, periosteal reaction)
Disease complications
● Angulation
● Ankylosis
● Malalignment
● Bone resorption
Soft tissue
● Swelling
● Effusion

Bones

Look at each bone in turn. First follow the cortical outline, then the internal trabecular pattern for disruption indicating a fracture (see 'Fractures', pp. 103–106, for
further characterization of fractures). Look for focal lesions (see 'Radiological characterization of bone lesions', pp. 106–109).

Joints

Check whether the joint spaces are even and parallel. Look for loose bodies within
a joint and calcification of articular cartilage. Familiarity with the common appearances of the athritides is important (see 'The radiology of joints', pp. 112–117).

Soft tissues

Identify any foreign bodies (e.g. glass), calcification, or gas or fluid levels within soft
tissues. Look for soft-tissue swelling, not only to help localize an underlying fracture,
but also to indicate a severe soft-tissue injury, such as knee effusion or ligament
tear. Remember that a fracture may be regarded as an osseous manifestation of a
serious soft-tissue injury.

━ **QUICK REFERENCE CHECKLIST** ━

Plain radiograph

Adequacy
Overview
Alignment
Bones
Joints
Soft tissues

Shoulder radiograph

The AP radiograph is supplemented by a further view, such as the axial, oblique axial or lateral. The axial and oblique axial necessitate arm abduction, which is not always possible if the shoulder is painful; therefore a lateral view is usually taken.

Overview

Bones

Review all the bones:

❑ humerus
❑ scapula
❑ clavicle
❑ ribs.

Humerus
For proximal humeral fractures (commonly through the surgical neck), note the number of fracture parts and the degree of displacement and angulation. Comment on the position of the articular head.

An impacted fracture of the posterolateral humeral head (Hill–Sachs lesion) may occur following anterior dislocation due to impaction of the humerus on the anterior glenoid.

Scapula
Do not miss subtle glenoid rim fractures, such as those of the antero-inferior glenoid following anterior dislocation (Bankart's fracture).

Joints

Glenohumeral joint
The humeral head should sit within the glenoid fossa and an even joint space should be maintained. An uneven joint space may be the only sign of posterior dislocation on the AP view.

Interpretation Tips

Shoulder radiograph

● When looking at the lateral, axial or oblique axial views, identify the coracoid process, which points anteriorly, as it will aid orientation.
● The 'light bulb sign' can be an unreliable indicator of posterior dislocation, as a normal humerus held in internal rotation will have this appearance. Therefore rely on the supplemental view to confirm posterior dislocation.
● Although osteoarthritis of the shoulder is rare, rheumatoid arthritis commonly affects the shoulder, indicated by periarticular osteopenia, cartilage loss and erosions (commonly of the acromioclavicular joint and superior lateral humeral head).
● If a clear fracture of the scapula is seen on the AP view, further attempts at plain radiography are unnecessary and painful. Go straight to CT with reformats.

QUICK REFERENCE CHECKLIST

Shoulder radiograph

Overview
Bones
● Humerus
● Scapula
● Clavicle
● Ribs
Joints
● Glenohumeral
● Acromioclavicular joint
Soft tissues
Lung

Anterior dislocation   Anterior dislocations are common. The humeral head overlaps the glenoid on the AP view and sits under the coracoid process inferomedial to the glenoid. On the supplemental view the humeral head is seen anterior to the glenoid fossa.

Posterior dislocation   Posterior dislocations can be subtle and must be actively sought. The AP view can look remarkably normal. Owing to internal rotation of the humerus following a posterior dislocation, the humeral head may have a 'light bulb' appearance. Supplemental views are crucial to confirm posterior dislocation, with the head of the humerus posterior to the glenoid fossa.

Acromioclavicular joint
The inferior border of the acromion should be aligned with the inferior border of the distal clavicle. Joint disruption leads to elevation of the distal clavicle (pulled by the

Fig. 6.8. Peri-articular calcification of the left shoulder, indicating degenerative joint disease.

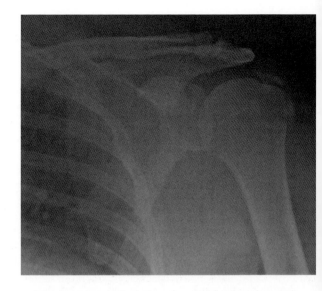

Fig. 6.9. The comminuted, displaced clavicle fracture is easy enough to spot, but fractures of the fifth and sixth ribs and apical pneumothorax are a little trickier.

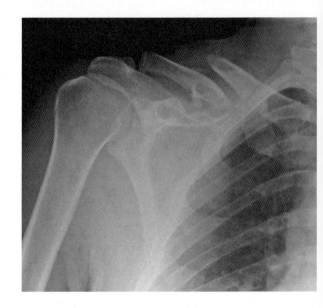

sternocleidomastoid muscle). Also look for widening (>10 mm) of the acromio-clavicular joint.

Soft tissues

Look for signs of rotator cuff pathology, such as a narrowed sub-acromial space (≤5 mm) and calcification (Fig. 6.8).

Lung

Do not forget to look for lung pathology, such as a pneumothorax or an incidental lung lesion (apical lung lesions are a recognized cause of shoulder pain) (Fig. 6.9).

Elbow radiograph

Standard views for elbow imaging are AP and lateral.

Overview

Alignment

Trace both the anterior humeral and the radiocapitellar line.

❏ *Anterior humeral line (lateral projection)*. Over a third of the capitellum should lie anterior to this line. If it does not, suspect a supracondylar fracture with posterior displacement of the distal fragments (Fig. 6.10).
❏ *Radiocapitellar line (lateral and AP projection)*. Trace a line through the centre of the proximal radius (see Fig. 6.10). This should pass through the capitellum; if it does not there is radial head dislocation (Fig. 6.11).

Bones

Often an impacted radial head fracture will manifest only as a transverse line of increased density, or a subtle buckle of the cortical outline.

Interpretation Tips

Elbow radiograph

● Elbow injuries in children are often difficult to interpret owing to multiple ossification centres (see Chapter 8).
● The most common cause of elevated fat pads following trauma, without an obvious bony abnormality, is an undisplaced radial head fracture.
● The absence of elevated fat pads does not exclude a fracture.
● Any cause of a large effusion from the elbow joint will elevate the fat pads (e.g. rheumatoid arthritis).
● The radius and ulna act as a bony ring; therefore, a fracture or dislocation of one bone will often lead to injury of the other.
● A dislocated radial head is associated with a displaced ulnar fracture (Monteggia injury). A displaced fracture of the proximal radius is associated with dislocation of the distal radioulnar joint (Galeazzi injury). Therefore, in the presence of any of these injuries in isolation, it is imperative to image the whole forearm and wrist.
● One way to remember which bone breaks is by remembering the sounds that a cow and a tiger make: MU (cow) – Monteggia = ulnar fracture; GR (tiger) – Galeazzi = radial fracture.

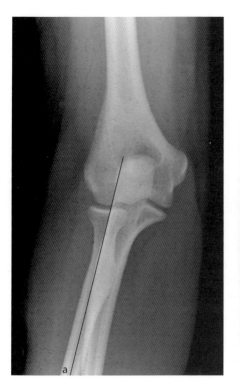

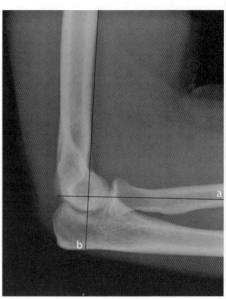

Fig. 6.10. Normal AP and lateral view of the right elbow. Ensure that the radius is in alignment with the capitellum on both views (a) and that at least one-third of the capitellum lies in front of the anterior humoral line (b).

Fig. 6.11. Dislocation of the radial head (compare with Fig. 6.10), often associated with an ulnar fracture (Monteggia injury).

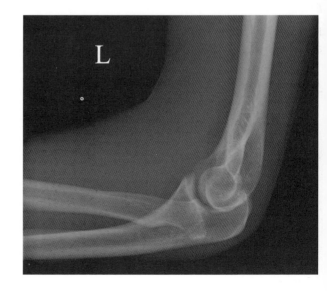

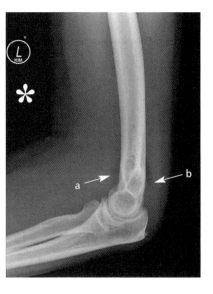

Fig. 6.12. Lateral view of the left elbow. There is elevation of the anterior (a) and posterior fat pads (b) signifying a joint effusion. In the context of trauma, this indicates a fracture until proven otherwise.

Fat pads

On the normal lateral view, the anterior fat pad is evident as thin lucency adjacent to the anterior cortical margin of the distal humeral diaphysis. An effusion will lift the anterior fat pad off the humerus and produces the appearance of a triangular lucency.

The posterior fat pad is not normally seen, and it should alert the observer to a fracture in the context of trauma (Fig. 6.12).

Elbow joint

Loose bodies within the elbow joint are often hidden within the olecranon fossa and are more apparent on the AP view.

Soft tissues

QUICK REFERENCE CHECKLIST

Elbow radiograph

Overview
Alignment
● Anterior humeral line
● Radiocapitellar line
Bones
Fat pads
Elbow joint
Soft tissues

Wrist radiograph

The wrist is prone to injury, particularly following a fall on an outstretched hand. Standard wrist views are dorsopalmar (DP) and lateral. If scaphoid injury is suspected, then two further supplemental views (oblique and dedicated scaphoid) are acquired.

Overview

Alignment

Familiarity with normal wrist alignment is the key to interpretation of the wrist radiograph. Joint spaces should be even and approximately 1–2 mm in width.

DP view

Three arcs can normally be traced around the carpal bones (Gilula's arcs, Fig. 6.13). If it is not possible to trace them, suspect carpal derangement.

Look for ulnar variance. Normally the distal ulna is a few millimetres shorter than the distal radius. If the ulna is over 2 mm longer than the radius, there is positive ulnar variance, indicating radial shortening, for example following a radial fracture.

Lateral view

On the lateral view, the radius, lunate and capitate should be aligned. Look for lunate (Fig. 6.14) and perilunate (Fig. 6.15) dislocation.

On a true lateral view, check the overlap of the radius and ulna: if they do not overlap, the distal radioulnar joint is dislocated.

Bones

Scaphoid and triquetral fractures make up the majority of carpal fractures; therefore it is vital to examine these bones thoroughly.

QUICK REFERENCE CHECKLIST

Wrist radiograph

Overview
Alignment
● DP
● Lateral
Bones
● Scaphiod
● Triquetral
● Lunate
Joints
Soft tissues

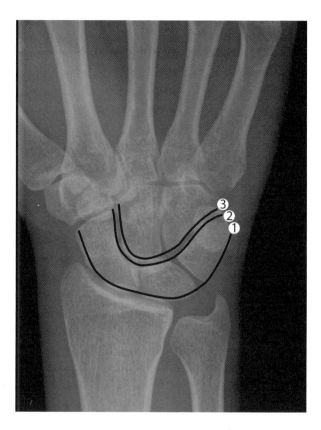

Fig. 6.13. Dorsopalmar (DP) view of the wrist with Gilula's arcs. Disruption of these arcs follows carpal subluxation or dislocation indicating carpal instability.

❏ *Scaphoid.* If injury is suspected, four scaphoid views are mandatory. The scaphoid is served by a blood supply entering from the distal pole; consequently, the proximal fragment is particularly prone to avascular necrosis following fracture. If a fracture is identified, record the location (i.e. proximal pole, distal pole or waist).

❏ *Triquetral.* On the lateral view of the wrist, a bone fragment seen dorsally over the carpal bones represents a triquetral fracture (Fig. 6.16).

Check the morphology of the lunate. A triangular appearance of the lunate on the AP view can indicate dislocation (see above). Repeated trauma to the lunate, for example from using a pneumatic drill, can lead to sclerosis and collapse of the lunate due to avascular necrosis (Kienböck's disease).

Joints

In addition to acute injury, chronic joint pathology may become apparent. Be aware of the radiographic appearances of common arthritides affecting the hand and wrist (see section on the hand radiograph and the interpretation tips, below).

Soft tissues

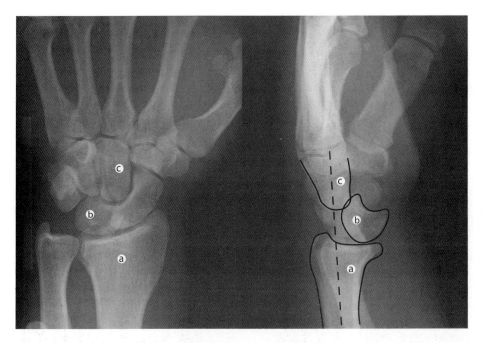

Fig. 6.14. Lunate dislocation and radial styloid fracture. Radius (a), lunate (b), capitate (c).

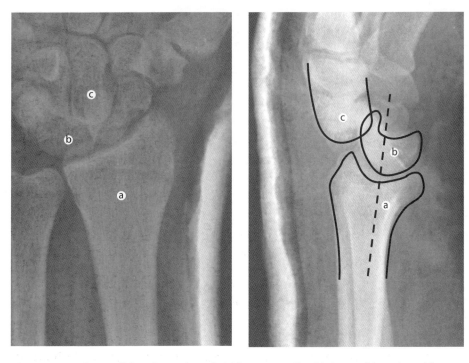

Fig. 6.15. Perilunate dislocation and scaphoid fracture. Radius (a), lunate (b), capitate (c).

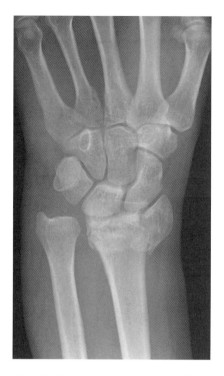
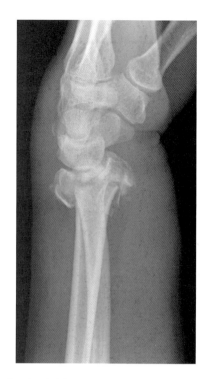

L

Fig. 6.16. Comminuted, impacted, intra-articular, left distal radial fracture with dorsal angulation and gross soft-tissue swelling. It is important to review the entire image as there is a small flake of bone dorsal to the distal carpal row on the lateral view, indicating an additional triquetral fracture.

Hand radiograph

Standard hand views for imaging the phalanges and metacarpals are the DP and oblique. Fingers are viewed with DP and lateral projections. Dedicated thumb views can also be acquired.

Overview

Bones

Look carefully for phalangeal avulsion fractures on the oblique or lateral views. These indicate either extensor tendon avulsion if dorsal (e.g. at the base of terminal phalanx resulting in a 'mallet finger' deformity) (Fig. 6.17), or volar plate injury if seen on the volar aspect of the phalanges. A peri-articular fragment of bone seen laterally on the DP view can indicate avulsion of a collateral ligament.

Joints

The joint spaces should be even. Ensure that there is no bone overlap, which would indicate dislocation. Pay particular attention to the carpometacarpal joints, which

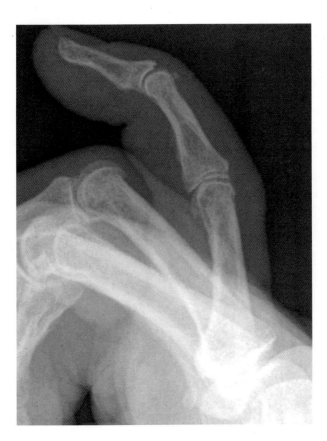

Fig. 6.17. Extensor tendon avulsion fracture at the base of the terminal phalanx – 'mallet finger'.

Interpretation Tips

Hand and wrist radiograph

- Dislocation of the carpometacarpal joints may be difficult to see on DP and oblique hand views, and is one of the few indications for a true lateral injury of the hand.
- Deformity without a fracture may indicate a tendon or ligament injury.
- Have a very low threshold for suspecting undisplaced scaphoid fracture, as missing this injury can result in considerable disability.
- Combination injuries of the wrist are common. For example, scaphoid fracture often accompanies perilunate dislocation, so do not be satisfied if only one injury is identified.
- Be aware of the common radiographic appearances of rheumatoid arthritis, osteoarthritis, calcium pyrophosphate arthropathy (pseudo-gout) and seronegative arthropathy (also see 'The radiology of joints', pp. 112–115).
- For rheumatoid arthritis, look for symmetrical erosive polyarthropathy predominantly affecting the metacarpophalangeal, proximal interphalangeal and intercarpal joints. Features include joint space narrowing, bone resorption, bone erosions, soft-tissue swelling and ankylosis

continued

Interpretation Tips continued

- For osteoarthritis, look for loss of joint space, subchondral sclerosis and osteophytes, particularly affecting the distal interphalangeal joints and the first carpometacarpal joint.
- Calcium pyrophosphate arthropathy preferentially affects the second and third metacarpophalangeal joints and first carpometacarpal joint. It is bilateral and symmetrical. It resembles osteoarthritis, but without involvement of the interphalangeal joints, with or without chondral calcification (of articular cartilage and the triangular fibrocartilage).
- Seronegative arthropathy results in erosions with maintained bone density affecting the whole chondral joint surface, not joint margins, with hyperostosis of the collateral insertions (unlike rheumatoid arthritis).

QUICK REFERENCE CHECKLIST

Hand radiograph

Overview
Alignment
Bones
Joints
Soft tissues
Carpal bones

should be 1–2 mm wide. Loss of this space, particularly of the fourth and fifth carpometacarpal joints, suggests a dislocation, which should be apparent on the oblique view.

Carpal bones

See 'Wrist radiograph', above.

Pelvis and hip radiograph

The dedicated pelvic radiograph is centred higher than a pelvis view taken specifically to look at the hips. Both should be reviewed in the same systematic way, as associated and incidental coexisting pathologies are common. If a hip fracture is suspected, a dedicated lateral hip view is also obtained.

Overview

Alignment

It is helpful to trace the lines detailed in Fig. 6.18 when checking alignment.

Femora

Look at each femoral head and neck in turn, checking for disruption of the trabecular pattern, which would indicate a subtle undisplaced fracture. If a femoral neck

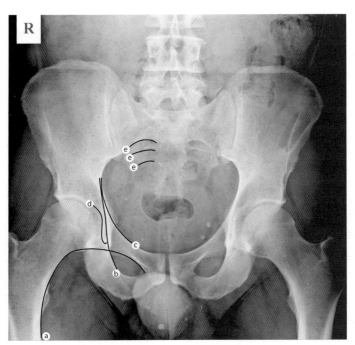

Fig. 6.18. AP pelvis demonstrating Shenton's line (a), ilioischial line (b), ileopectineal line (c), teardrop line (d) and the sacral foramina (e) on the right. Note the lucent lesion within the left iliac wing, representing a renal carcinoma metastasis (see Fig. 6.20). Note that this lucency lies outside the line of the descending colon and should not be confused with bowel gas.

fracture is identified, comment on the location and degree of displacement. Femoral neck fractures are divided into intracapsular or extracapsular, as this classification determines management:

❏ Intracapsular fractures, which represent two-thirds of hip fractures, are liable to avascular necrosis, due to disruption of the retinacular artery.
❏ The proximal femur remains well vascularized in extracapsular fractures; there-fore avascular necrosis is unlikely (<1% of cases).

Check that the femoral head is smooth and rounded within the acetabulum.

Hip joint

The hip joint should be smooth and even. Comment on any arthritic changes (see 'The radiology of joints', pp. 112–115).

Acetabula

Scrutinize the acetabula closely following trauma as fractures here are easily missed. Look for disruption of the iliopectineal, ilioischial and teardrop lines (see Fig. 6.18).

Pubic rami, ischia and symphysis

Check both the superior and the inferior pubic rami and ischia for fractures and lesions. Look for widening or overlapping of the symphysis.

Interpretation Tips

Pelvis and hip radiograph

- If a fracture of the pelvis is seen, look hard for a second fracture, as the pelvis is a bony ring and likely to fracture in two places, representing an unstable injury. Associated visceral injury is common.
- Beware of subtle, undisplaced impacted fractures of the femoral neck, which may manifest as a line of sclerosis that does not traverse the entire femoral neck. If doubt remains, or the clinical suspicion is high, further imaging may be needed (e.g. bone scan or MRI).
- Subtrochanteric fractures are frequently pathological; therefore look carefully for evidence of metastases, myeloma or Paget's disease elsewhere on the radiograph.
- Identifying fractures in the presence of extensive ring osteophytes in osteoarthritis can be challenging, as they can be mistaken for a fracture line. If spurs are seen on the lateral and medial margins, a fracture is unlikely. If in doubt, recommend further imaging.
- Overlying bowel gas may produce false bone 'lucency'; likewise, lytic bone lesions may be misinterpreted as overlying gas (see Figs 6.18 and 6.20).

Iliac wings

Look at each iliac wing, being mindful of common bony pelvic pathologies, such as:

- ❏ *Paget's disease* – increased bone density with a coarsened tarbecular pattern (Fig. 6.19)
- ❏ *malignancy* – focal decreased density of myeloma and lytic metastases, or focal increased density of sclerotic metastases (Fig. 6.20).

Sacroiliac joints

Comment on any loss of definition of the cortical margins of the sacroiliac joints, sclerosis, erosions or joint space narrowing. Identify any ankylosis of the joint. Describe the distribution of the changes:

- ❏ bilateral and symmetrical (e.g. ankylosing spondylitis)
- ❏ bilateral and asymmetrical (e.g. rheumatoid arthritis)
- ❏ unilateral (e.g. infection).

Sacrum

Check that the sacral foramina are even and clearly defined and that no sacral fractures are present (see Fig. 6.18).

Avulsion fractures

Look specifically for avulsion injuries following trauma:

Fig. 6.19. AP view of the pelvis demonstrating a coarsened trabecular pattern of the right ilium, ischium and pubis typical of Paget's disease. There are also secondary degenerative changes within the right hip in addition to degenerative appearances in the lower lumbar spine.

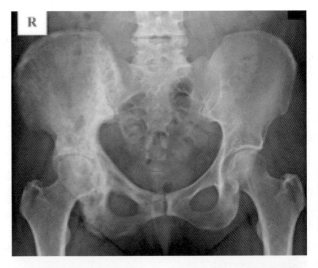

Fig. 6.20. The same patient as in Fig. 6.18, 8 months later, now demonstrating a large lytic metastasis in the left iliac wing secondary to metastatic renal carcinoma.

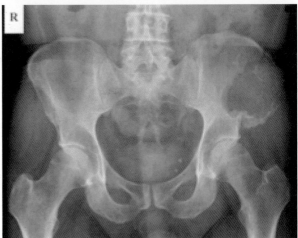

- ❏ greater trochanter–gluteus medius (common after a fall)
- ❏ lesser trochanter–iliopsoas (rare and often with a sinister pathological cause)
- ❏ anterosuperior iliac spine–sartorius
- ❏ anteroinferior iliac spine–rectus femoris (commoner in athletes)
- ❏ ischial tuberosity – (hamstrings).

Lumbar spine

It is important not to miss gross spinal pathology.

Soft tissues

Finally, check the pelvic soft tissues and note any calcification (e.g. phleboliths, bladder calculi, calcified fibroids) or abnormal bowel gas pattern.

Knee radiograph

Standard knee views are the AP and lateral (horizontal beam lateral following trauma). The patello-femoral articulation is best seen on a skyline view and loose bodies within the intercondylar notch are identified on a tunnel view.

Overview

Effusion

Study the horizontal lateral view for a simple effusion or a lipohaemarthrosis within the suprapatellar bursa. On the lateral view there should be less than a 5 mm depth of fluid in the suprapatella bursa; any more indicates an effusion.

Tibial plateau and tibia

Tibial plateau fractures can be very subtle and are easily overlooked. The lateral plateau is most often injured as the lateral femoral condyle is driven downwards following a twisting or side-impact injury. Pay attention to alignment on the AP image, and check that the lateral edges of the tibial plateaus and femoral condyles align: if the plateau overhangs, suspect a fracture. Remember, most tibial plateau fractures involve the articular surface, but usually spare the rim. Look at both the AP and lateral views for subtle irregularities; sclerotic horizontal density on the AP view below the plateau signifies an impacted fragment (Figs 6.21 and 6.22).

Joint space

Look for focal and global loss of joint space. Acute loss of joint space can occur following trauma or chronically as a sign of degenerative or chronic inflammatory change. Search hard for calcified loose bodies within the knee; these could be fracture fragments or avulsed ligamentous insertions.

Fibular head

Fractures of the fibular head are rarely isolated findings, and if identified look again for subtle tibial plateau fractures. Also, have a high index of suspicion for significant ligamentous injury or even an associated tibial or ankle fracture.

Femur

Follow the cortex of the femur, paying particular attention to the femoral condyles on the AP view for osteochondral fractures of the articular surface. For supracondylar fractures, record whether there is intra-articular extension; if not, record the distance from the fracture to the joint space.

Patella

First look for fractures, best seen on the AP view, being careful not to confuse a break with a bipartite patella. The smaller component of a bipartite patella is frequently situated superolaterally and the bony margins are corticated.

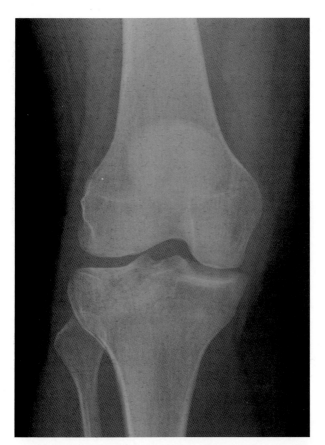

Fig. 6.21. AP view of a lateral tibial plateau fracture: disordered trabecular pattern and a double lateral tibial plateau border.

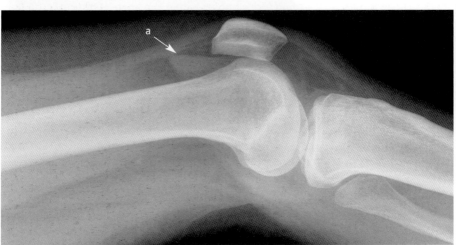

Fig. 6.22. Lateral view of the same joint as in Fig. 6.21. The presence of a lipohaemarthrosis (a) within the suprapatella bursa on the horizontal beam lateral image confirms an intra-articular fracture.

QUICK REFERENCE CHECKLIST

Pelvis and hip radiograph

Overview
Alignment
Femora
Hip joint
Acetabula
Pubic rami, ischia and symphysis
Iliac wings
Sacroiliac joints
Sacrum
Avulsion fractures
Lumbar spine
Soft tissues

Then check that the alignment of the patella is satisfactory and that it is not laterally placed. Beware that the only sign of a recent patella dislocation may be a small effusion. Comment on the height of the patella if this is abnormal: 'patella alta' is high riding and 'patella baja' is low riding (either a longstanding finding or a sign of rupture of the patella tendon or quadriceps tendon, respectively).

Soft tissues

Finally, scrutinize the soft tissues for pathology such as a mass within the popliteal fossa (e.g. Baker's cyst) or gas within the soft tissues in the context of a compound fracture or gas-forming infection.

Interpretation Tips

Knee radiograph

- Beware that severe meniscal and ligamentous injury can occur in the absence of a fracture.
- Subtle tibial plateau fractures can be hard to detect on the plain film, so have a high index of suspicion.
- A small lateral avulsion fragment is often associated with injury to the anterior cruciate ligament and meniscal injury (Segond fracture – Fig. 6.23).
- Have a high index of suspicion for associated fractures, even at the ankle, when an apparently isolated fracture of the fibular head is seen. Damage to the common peroneal nerve often accompanies such a fracture.

Fig. 6.23. Segond facture. The seemingly trivial fracture fragment seen lateral to the tibia (a) is frequently associated with injury to the anterior cruciate ligament and meniscal injury.

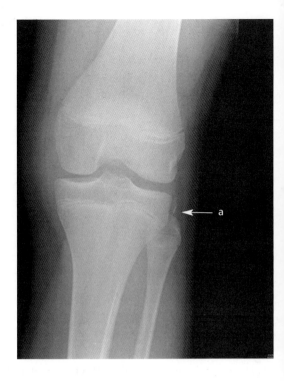

QUICK REFERENCE CHECKLIST

Knee radiograph

Overview
Effusion
Tibial plateau and tibia
Joint space
Fibular head
Femur
Patella
Soft tissues

Ankle radiograph

The ankle acts as a bony and ligamentous ring, and the talus is located within this ring in a compound fossa (Fig. 6.24). Therefore, when a fracture is identified at one site, it is likely that there has been another injury (either bone or ligamentous) at another site within the ring. Note also that injuries of the ankle and foot, covered in the next section, often occur in association.

Standard views of the ankle are an AP and lateral.

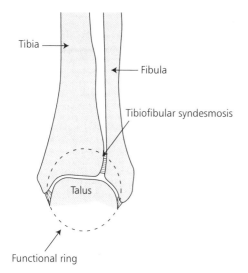

Fig. 6.24. Functional ring of the ankle joint.

Tibia

Fibula

Tibiofibular syndesmosis

Talus

Functional ring

Overview

AP view

Alignment

Check the position of the talus. The talotibial and talofibular joint spaces should be uniform. Asymmetrical widening of the joint space in the absence of a fracture suggests a potentially unstable ligamentous disruption of the functional ring.

Bones

Look at the contour of the talar dome, and for evidence of cortical irregularity. Osteochondral defects are common here and can lead to secondary osteoarthritis of the joint.

Look for evidence of a fracture of either the medial or lateral malleolus. If the lateral malleolus (fibula) is fractured, then note the position of the fracture in relation to the tibio-fibular syndesmosis. This is the basis of the Weber classification of ankle fractures and has important implications for joint stability and surgical intervention.

Soft tissues

Lateral view

Check that the projection is true lateral: the fibula and tibia should overlap and the base of the fifth metatarsal should be included.

Alignment

Check the position of the talus. If the projection is true lateral, the fibula should overlap the talar dome. If not, suspect a talar dislocation.

137

Bones

Look for a fracture of the posterior malleolus. An oblique fracture of the posterior distal tibia can be subtle and represents a potentially unstable injury, so look carefully.

Look through the tibia at the fibula. Oblique fractures of the fibula can be invisible on the AP view and seen only on the lateral view.

Soft tissues

> **Interpretation Tip**
>
> **Ankle radiograph**
>
> ● Because of the various ligament attachments, small avulsion fractures are common. In particular, check the base of the fifth metatarsal bone (Fig. 6.25).

Fig. 6.25. Review areas on the lateral ankle radiograph: posterior malleolus (a), fibula (b), anterior lip of tibia (c), calcaneus (d), anterior process of calcaneus (e), superior aspect of talonavicular joint (f) and fractures of the base of the fifth metatarsal, as demonstrated here (g). Bohler's angle is also demonstrated, which should not be <30°.

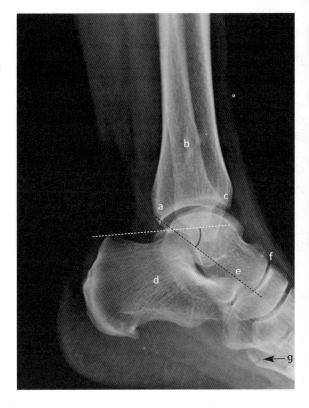

Ankle radiograph

Overview
AP view
● Alignment
 – Widening of joint space in the ankle mortice
● Bones
 – Defects of the talar dome
 – Medial and lateral malleoli
● Soft tissues
Lateral view
● Alignment
 – Talus
● Bones
 – Posterior malleolus
 – Look at the fibula through the tibia
● Soft tissues
● Review areas (see Fig. 6.25)

Foot radiograph

The most common projections of the foot are a dorsoplantar view and an oblique view. These, however, do not adequately demonstrate all bones of the foot (e.g. cuboid and navicular). If a calcaneal injury is suspected, dedicated calcaneal projections are necessary.

Overview
Alignment

Lisfranc fracture dislocations are uncommon but highly important foot injuries that can cause considerable disability if not treated early. They comprise a variable spectrum of foot fractures and/or dislocations around the Lisfranc joints (the tarsometatarsal joints) between the mid-foot and forefoot (Figs 6.26 and 6.27).

Midtarsal joints
A wavy (S-shaped) line at the midtarsal joint (the joint separating the talus and calcaneus from the navicular and cuboid, respectively) should be intact, thus confirming the integrity of this joint (see Fig. 6.26).

Bones

Assess each bone for evidence of a fracture. Stress fractures can be very subtle.

Calcaneal fractures often result from a fall from a height causing axial loading and are therefore associated with fractures of the pelvis and spinal column. Check for

Fig. 6.26. Normal alignment of the Lisfranc joints (a) and the midtarsal joints (b).

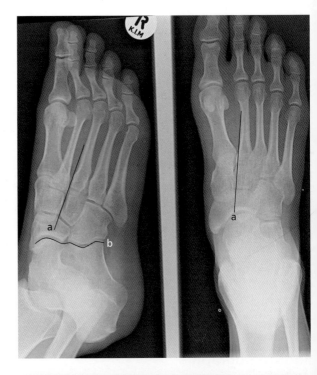

Fig. 6.27. Lisfranc fracture, in addition to a spiral fracture of the third metatarsal.

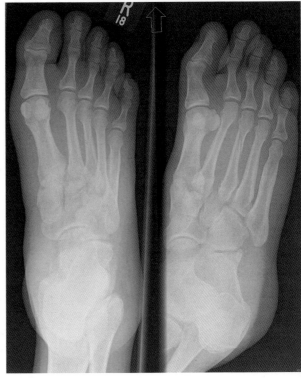

evidence of a fracture. The only evidence may be a line of sclerosis or interruption of trabeculation.

Compression fractures may result in a reduced Bohler's angle (<30°) (see Fig. 6.25).

Soft tissues

> ### Interpretation Tips
>
> **Foot radiograph**
>
> ● A Lisfranc injury may show delayed displacement and therefore be radiographically occult. The gold standard for demonstrating a Lisfranc injury is a weight-bearing dorsoplantar view.
> ● There are a number of ossicles usually in characteristic locations that should not be confused with avulsion fractures, and reference to an atlas of normal variants is useful here.

> **QUICK REFERENCE CHECKLIST**
>
> Overview
> Alignment
> ● Lisfranc lines
> ● Midtarsal joints
> Bones
> ● Calcaneum
> ● Soft tissues

APPENDICULAR MRI

Shoulder MRI

MRI, with its excellent discrimination between soft tissue and bone, is ideally suited to characterizing pathology of the rotator cuff. It can also be used to assess arthritis, infection and neoplastic disorders of the shoulder.

Imaging protocols vary between centres. The primary imaging plane is coronal oblique, acquired along the axis of the blade of the scapula; therefore slices are perpendicular to the glenoid. Sagittal oblique images are acquired at 90° to coronal oblique slices.

Protocols invariably include a coronal oblique T1-weighted sequence and a coronal oblique water-sensitive sequence (STIR, PD fat sat or gradient T2*). Most centres will also acquire a fat-suppressed sagittal oblique sequence (PD fat sat, fat sat T2 or STIR) and an axial sequence (e.g. PD fat sat). Sagittal T1-weighted scans are also acquired in some centres.

Overview

Scan the images for gross pathology (e.g. displaced fractures, large effusions and oedema) before conducting a thorough systematic search.

Bones

Look for:

❏ marrow oedema (coronal oblique water-sensitive sequence)
❏ cortical defects (e.g. Hill–Sachs or glenoid lesions) (coronal T1-weighted sequence)
❏ osteophytes and erosions (coronal T1-weighted sequence)
❏ subacromial bone spurs (associated with shoulder impingement syndrome and rotator cuff tears) (coronal T1-weighted sequence)
❏ presence of an os acromiale (an unfused lateral acromion), which may be unstable and is associated with impingement and rotator cuff tears (axial sequence)
❏ abnormality of the joint space of the glenohumoral and acromioclavicular joints (water-sensitive sequences).

Synovium

Look for an effusion within the glenohumoral joint and fluid within the subacromial bursa. A high-signal connection between the two implies a full-thickness tear of the rotator cuff. Identify any filling defects (loose bodies) within the glenohumoral joint (coronal oblique water-sensitive sequence).

Rotator cuff

The rotator cuff provides stability to the glenohumoral joint along with the glenoid labrum and the glenohumoral ligament. Rotator cuff tears are common, and acute tears show as areas of increased signal intensity on water-sensitive sequences. Individually check each muscle for fluid signal crossing the fibres, indicating a tear. Ensure that each segment is seen in at least two planes:

❏ Supraspinatus – coronal and sagittal oblique
❏ Infraspinatus, subscapularis and teres minor – sagittal oblique and axial.

On the coronal T1 images look for additional secondary signs of rotator cuff pathology:

❏ muscle atrophy
❏ fatty muscle replacement
❏ retraction of muscle and tendon fibres
❏ wavy contour of muscle fibres.

Figs 6.28–6.31 compare intact and torn supraspinatus and subscapularis muscles and tendons.

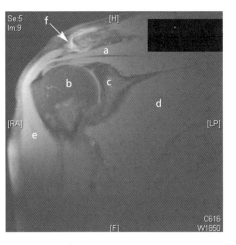

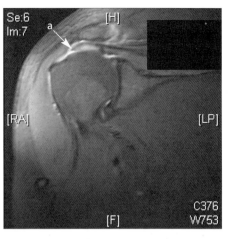

Fig. 6.28. Coronal oblique T2-weighted image showing the intact supraspinatus muscle and tendon (a). Humoral head (b), glenoid (c), subscapularis (d), deltoid (e). Note the incidental high signal around the acromioclavicular joint (f).

Fig. 6.29. Coronal oblique STIR image of a supraspinatus tear – compare with Fig. 6.28. The tendon has retracted (a) and is surrounded by high-signal fluid.

Long head of biceps

Check that the long head of biceps lies within the bicipital groove. Ensure that it is not thickened, split or surrounded with fluid (normal diameter is 3–5 mm).

Pay particular attention to the 'anterior interval'. This is the area, best seen on axial and sagittal images, traversed by the long head of biceps between supraspinatus anteriorly and subscapularis. This is a common site of synovitis, impingement and tears.

Review areas

Finally, check:

❏ the axilla for mass lesions or lymphadenopathy
❏ the suprascapular notch, as lesions here can cause shoulder pain due to impingement on the suprascapular nerve.

Interpretation Tips

Shoulder MRI

● The long head of biceps can be bifid within the groove as a normal variant
● The supraspinatus tendon is the commonest site for rotator cuff tears.

continued

Fig. 6.30. Axial view of the right subscapularis muscle and tendon (a). Humoral head (b), glenoid (c), infraspinatus (d) and deltoid (e).

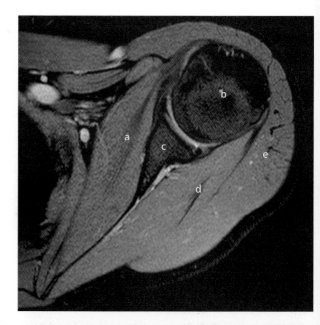

Fig. 6.31. Subscapularis tear – compare with Fig. 6.30. Axial proton density (PD)-weighted fat-suppressed MR scan of the left shoulder demonstrating retraction of the tendon (a) and high signal within the muscle itself (b).

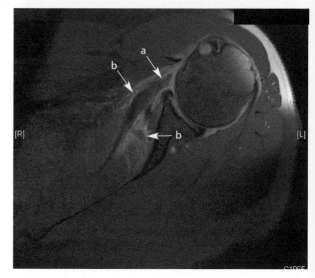

Interpretation Tips *continued*

- Chronic rotator cuff tears may be difficult to detect as they may not display relative high intensity on water-sensitive sequences. Look for the secondary signs of rotator cuff injury such as muscle atrophy and retraction.
- Tears of the glenoid labrum are not well appreciated on MRI unless they are large, seen as an area of increased signal. MR arthrography is required to accurately characterize labral tears.

> **QUICK REFERENCE CHECKLIST**
>
> **Shoulder MRI**
>
> Overview
> Bones
> Synovium
> Rotator cuff
> Long head of biceps
> Review areas
> ● Axilla
> ● Suprascapular notch

Knee MRI

MRI is the primary imaging modality to characterize soft tissue, ligamentous and cartilaginous derangement of the knee. The role of CT is largely confined to characterizing the number and position of bone fragments following a complex fracture. In addition to trauma, referral indications for MRI include ongoing knee pain, locking, swelling and tumour.

Of the sequences, T2-weighted images provide the most information, as the synovial fluid outlines the internal knee architecture with high 'white' signal.

Tendons and ligaments display a uniform low signal on T1- and T2-weighted sequences. Tears are identified as either interruption of the fibres or focal higher-signal areas of oedema and haemorrhage, particularly on T2-weighted images.

The protocol in our centre is:

- ❏ T1 sagittal
- ❏ T2* (gradient echo) sagittal and coronal (standard T2-weighted images can also be used)
- ❏ proton density (PD) fat saturation axial if pathology is suspected in the anterior compartment
- ❏ short-tau inversion recovery (STIR) if after trauma.

Other protocols include three-dimensional PD-weighted and sagittal or coronal PD fat saturation.

Overview

- ❏ Sagittal and coronal T2*/T2.

Start with a global overview looking at the alignment of the knee joint. Note any large effusions, filling defects or loose bodies within the knee joint. Note whether the medial and lateral joint spaces are preserved. Look for the plicae – synovial remnants within the knee joint found within 60% of normal individuals, which appear as linear intermediate signal within the knee joint.

Cruciate ligaments

❑ Sagittal T1 and T2*/T2.

Anterior cruciate ligament
The anterior cruciate ligament runs from anterior to the tibial intercondylar eminence to the medial aspect of the lateral femoral condyle (Fig. 6.32). It looks thin, but is extremely strong. Tears are most common in the mid-substance and avulsions are usually from the femoral attachment (Fig. 6.33). The anterior edge should be taught and straight; posterior bowing can indicate a chronic tear.

Posterior cruciate ligament
The posterior cruciate ligament runs from the lateral aspect of the medial femoral condyle to the posterior intercondylar fossa of the tibia. It is thicker and darker than the anterior cruciate ligament. Again, tears occur most frequently within the mid-substance, and avulsions occur at its tibial insertion. Complete tears manifest as a gap in the ligament.

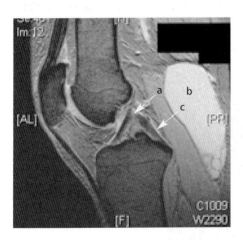 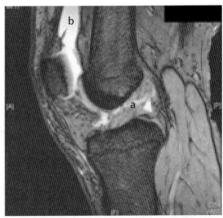

Fig. 6.32. Sagittal T2-weighted MR scan of a normal anterior cruciate ligament (a). There is also a large Baker's cyst within the popliteal fossa (b). The distal part of the posterior cruciate ligament is also seen on this section (c).

Fig. 6.33. Compare with Fig. 6.32. Instead of a thin, low-signal anterior cruciate ligament, the fibres are obscured by intermediate/high signal representing a grade III tear (a). Note the associated effusion within the suprapatella bursa (b).

Menisci

❏ Sagittal and coronal T1 and T2*/T2.

These C-shaped fibrocartilages sit on the condylar surface of the tibia, aiding mechanical stability of the knee. They are triangular in cross-section and display a homogeneous low signal. They should be intact in all planes with crisp, tapered margins.

Displaced longitudinal tears are referred to as 'bucket handle' tears. Increased signal on T2-weighted images due to imbibed synovial fluid indicates a tear (Fig. 6.34). Increased signal not communicating with the articular surface can indicate degenerative change (intra-substance high signal near the periphery of the meniscus is normal in children and teenagers).

Cysts (rounded low-signal areas on T1-weighted scans and high-signal areas on T2-weighted scans) within the meniscus can be secondary to degeneration or trauma.

Subchondral marrow oedema

❏ All planes, marrow sensitive sequences.

Displaced fractures will be evident on all planes and sequences. Use the sequences that are sensitive to marrow oedema (i.e. PD fat sat or STIR) to look for subtle increased signal within the bone, which will indicate a microtrabecular fracture, also known as 'bone bruising' (Fig. 6.35).

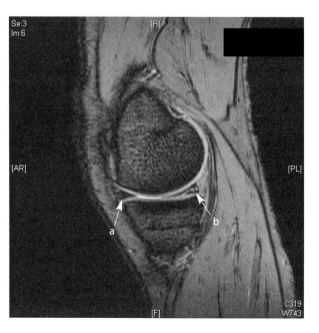

Fig. 6.34. Sagittal T2-weighted MRI demonstrating a medial meniscus tear. Compare the normal low-signal anterior horn of the medial meniscus (a) with the posterior horn of the medial meniscus. The tear appears as a line of high signal within the meniscus (b).

Fig. 6.35. STIR image demonstrating marrow oedema within the lateral femoral condyle.

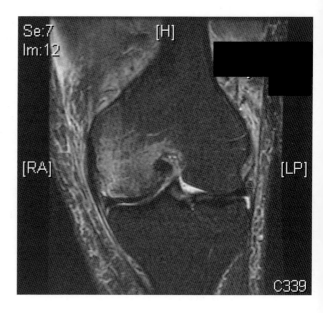

Collateral ligaments

❏ Coronal T1 and T2*/T2.

Medial collateral ligament

The medial collateral ligament runs from the medial femoral epicondyle to 5 cm below the medial tibial plateau. Signs of injury include increased distance between the subcutaneous tissues and bone, and increased signal on T2-/T2*-weighted images of haemorrhage and oedema around the fibres. Complete tears are associated with large joint effusions. Chronic injury to the ligament can result in thickening, with no increase in signal.

Lateral collateral ligament

The lateral collateral ligament is extracapsular and runs from the biceps femoris tendon to the fibular head. Injuries are rarer and harder to detect than those of the medial collateral ligament. Again, the ligament is low signal and damage is associated with increased signal on T2-weighted sequences.

Anterior compartment

❏ Axial T2* and T2; PD fat sat; sagittal T1 and T2.

The anterior compartment consists of the quadriceps tendon, patella, patellofemoral joint and the patella tendon.

Quadriceps tendon

Oedema and haemorrhage appear as high signal within the tendon. Look for fraying of the muscle fibres. A retracted proximal or distal muscle bundle can sometimes be observed as a soft-tissue mass with higher intensity than the surrounding muscle. Coronal and sagittal images can be useful to evaluate the extent of muscle involvement.

Patella and patellofemoral joint
Check that the patella is correctly aligned between the condyles. Look at the articular cartilage on the medial and lateral facets of the patella for thinning and high signal of oedema (axial images are required for cartilage assessment). Check the integrity of the medial and lateral retinacular attachments and marrow oedema within the patella itself.

Patella tendon
Check the integrity of the tendon from its insertion on the tibial tubercle to the patella. Look for tears and abnormal thickening which can occur following trauma.

Popliteal fossa
❏ Axial T1 and T2*/T2.

Conclude the review by checking for common pathology within the popliteal fossa, such as a Baker's cysts or a popliteal artery aneurysm (see Fig. 6.32).

Interpretation Tips

Knee MRI

- If an abnormality is seen in one plane, look in another to confirm the findings.
- Posterior and anterior to the posterior cruciate ligament are the ligaments of Wrisburg and Humphrey, respectively. These are normal structures and should not be confused with torn ligamentous fibres.
- If a ligamentous tear is identified, grade the injury: I = <25%; II = >25%; III = complete.
- Articular extension of meniscal tears can be hard to identify, so look for associated signs of injury (e.g. effusion) if a tear is suspected.
- A displaced meniscal fragment may come to rest within the intercondylar notch and sometimes gives the impression of a second posterior cruciate ligament – the so-called 'pseudo posterior cruciate ligament' sign.
- Do not mistake flow void within vessels for clot.

QUICK REFERENCE CHECKLIST

Knee MRI

Overview
Cruciate ligaments
Menisci
Subchondral marrow oedema
Collateral ligaments
Anterior compartment
Popliteal fossa

SPINAL IMAGING

Cervical spine radiograph

The cervical spine radiograph is a notoriously challenging investigation to interpret, because of the complex three-dimensional anatomy. Relatively inexperienced trainees should not expect to identify every subtle film abnormality; rather, they should aim to identify potential abnormalities requiring a more experienced opinion. In trauma it is helpful to regard the plain film, along with the history (high- or low-risk injury), as a screening tool to decide which patients require imaging with CT or MRI. For further reference see the 2007 guidelines on cervical spine trauma from the National Institute for Health and Clinical Excellence (available at www.nice.org.uk/CG56).

Adequacy

Standard views are the lateral, peg and AP:

❏ *Lateral*. The C7–T1 junction must be seen. If it is not, request a repeat with the arms pulled down or an additional 'swimmer's view'.
❏ *Peg view*. Check for rotation using the mandible for reference. The C1–C2 articulation and the peg should be visible.
❏ *AP view*. Check that the image is not rotated (as shown by equidistance of the medial ends of the clavicles from the spinous process) and that the entire cervical spine is included.

Overview

Display all the images together and review for gross pathology and malalignment before scrutinizing each image in turn.

Lateral view

Skull base, C1, C2
Check for craniocervical dissociation and the relation of the peg to the anterior arch of C1 (Fig. 6.36).

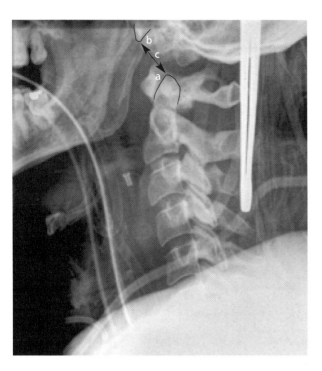

Fig. 6.36. The peg (a) normally sits beneath the clivus (b). The distance between the two should be ≤12 mm. In this case the distance between the two is grossly increased (c), indicating craniocervical dissociation.

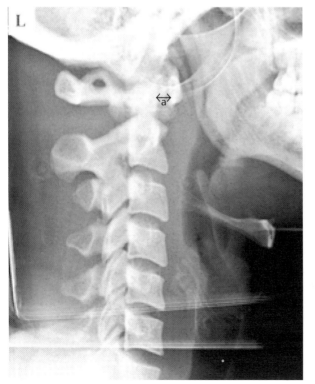

Fig. 6.37. C1 burst fracture. Note the increased distance between the peg and the anterior arch of C1 (a) and the associated soft-tissue swelling.

Fig. 6.38. Normal lateral cervical spine radiograph with anterior vertebral (a), posterior vertebral (b) and spinolaminar lines (c) marked. The rhomboid facet joints of C3 and C4 are outlined (d).

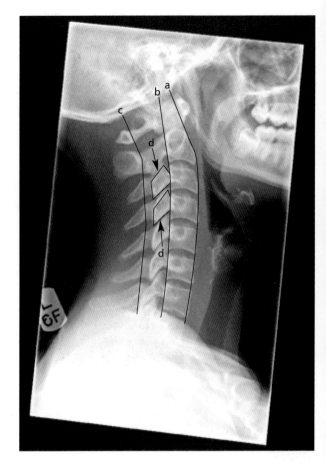

Look for C1 and C2 fractures. Check that the distance between the anterior aspect of the peg and the posterior aspect of the anterior arch of C1 is ≤3 mm in adults and ≤5 mm in children (Fig. 6.37).

Alignment
Ensure satisfactory alignment by tracing the anterior vertebral, posterior vertebral and spinolaminar lines (Fig. 6.38).

A general rule is that if the degree of forward vertebral slip is less than 25% of vertebral body width, there is likely to be unifacet dislocation; if it is more than 50%, then bifacet dislocation is likely.

Vertebrae
Check that vertebral body height is preserved and look for disruption of the cortical margin.

Look for fragments of bone anteriorly and inferiorly (teardrop fracture). Even though these can be small, they can indicate a serious hyperflexion injury.

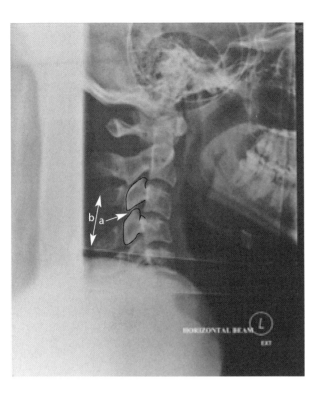

Fig. 6.39. Loss of parallel alignment of the C3–C4 facets (a) and splaying of the spinous processes (b) due to hyperflexion injury.

Disc spaces and facet joints

Ensure that the disc spaces are an even height and check the facet joint margins are equal and parallel (Figs 6.38 and 6.39).

Soft tissues

Look for prevertebral soft-tissue swelling. Normal prevertebral soft tissue is <7 mm wide for C1–4 and 22 mm for C5–7.

Identify any foreign bodies (e.g. venous lines, endotracheal tube).

Peg view

Alignment

The C1 and C2 lateral masses should align; if C1 overhangs C2, this is indicative of a burst fracture of C1. Check that the distance between the peg and the C1 body each side is even (beware, as this may be simulated by rotation, but there will not be overhang of C1 on C2 if this is just rotational) (Fig. 6.40).

Outline

Follow the outline of the peg and the remainder of C2 and C1, checking for fractures.

Ensure that the joint space between C1 and C2 is even and parallel.

Fig. 6.40. Peg view of a C1 burst fracture. The left lateral margin of C1 and C2 do not align (a), and the distance between the peg and the medial margin of C1 is increased (b).

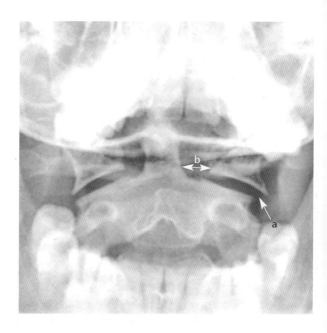

AP view

Alignment
Check that the spinous processes are approximately equidistant (more than 150% of the space above or below suggests anterior dislocation) and are in alignment (if not, consider unifacet dislocation as a cause of vertebral body rotation and malalignment).

Lateral masses
Carefully follow down one set of lateral masses, then the other, looking for fractures.

Joints
Check that the disc spaces are even and the end-plates parallel.

Soft tissues
Look for soft-tissue swelling, foreign bodies and displacement of the laryngeal and tracheal air column.

Lung apices
Look for incidental lung lesions, pneumothoraces, cervical ribs and rib fractures.

Interpretation Tips

Cervical spine radiograph

● Injuries to the lower cervical spine are common; it is therefore vital to image the entirety of the cervical spine.
● Extensive spondylitic changes in elderly people (e.g. osteophytes and facet joint subluxation) can render interpretation difficult; therefore have a low threshold for further imaging with CT.
● Prevertebral soft-tissue swelling is frequently not evident, even following fracture, so do not be falsely reassured by its absence.
● Beware of overlapping structures, such as the incisors and the occiput, which can give the false impression of a peg fracture, although fracture lines will not extend beyond the margins of the peg.
● Rotation of the T1 and T2 spinous processes on the AP view can be a normal finding.
● The key to interpreting the 'swimmer's view' is to identify the first rib of the elevated arm to identify the T1–C7 junction and work up from this point.
● The upper cervical spinous processes are bifid and it is important when checking alignment on the AP view to use the centres of the bifid processes, as uneven bifid processes can give the false impression of malalignment.

QUICK REFERENCE CHECKLIST

Cervical spine radiograph

Adequacy
Overview
Lateral view
● Skull base, C1, C2
● Alignment
● Vertebrae
● Disc spaces and facet joints
● Soft tissues
Peg view
● Alignment
● Outline
 – Joint space
AP view
● Alignment
● Lateral masses
● Joints
● Soft tissues
● Lung apices

Thoracic and lumbar spine radiograph

Degenerative, osteoporotic and metastatic pathology is frequently detected.

Lateral view

Alignment
Comment on any loss of alignment after tracing the anterior and posterior vertebral lines. Forward slip of one vertebra on another (spondylolisthesis) may indicate:

❑ facet joint osteoarthritis
❑ a defect in the pars interarticularis (that part of the posterior elements seen on the lateral view between the superior or inferior articular facets)
❑ a fracture.

Check that the normal mild thoracic kyphosis and lumbar lordosis are maintained.

Vertebrae
Comment on the overall bone quality. Look at each vertebra in turn, checking that the height and shape are maintained. Check that the margins of each vertebra are smooth and no erosions are present. Particularly following trauma, check for wedge fractures, and fractures of the posterior elements. Look for retropulsed fragments within the spinal canal.

In traumatic spinal injury, divide the spine into three columns: anterior, middle and posterior (Fig. 6.41). Any injury involving two or more columns should be regarded as unstable. An injury to the middle column is inherently unstable.

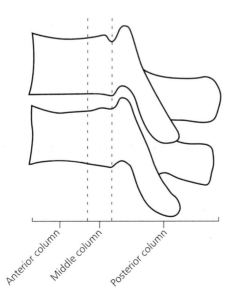

Anterior column

Middle column

Posterior column

Fig. 6.41. Three-column model of spinal stability. Any injury involving two or more columns should be regarded as unstable. An injury to the middle column is inherently unstable.

Disc spaces
Note any focal loss (or, rarely, increase) in disc space height. Disc space narrowing is most often degenerative in aetiology.

AP view

Alignment
If a scoliosis is present, describe the side to which there is convexity.

Check the alignment of:

❏ lateral aspects of the vertebral bodies
❏ pedicles (seen as 'owl's eyes' on the AP view)
❏ spinous processes.

Vertebrae
Vertebral bodies   Assess the height and shape of each vertebra.

Pedicles   Ensure that the pedicles are clearly defined. Widening of the pedicles at one level can indicate a burst fracture. Loss of definition of a pedicle often signifies bone destruction by malignancy (Figs 6.42 and 6.43).

Spinous processes   The spinous processes are not well seen on the lateral view, so on the AP view check the integrity of each process and that the interspinous distance is even.

Disc spaces
Again, check that all the disc spaces are even in height.

Paraspinal tissues
Carefully trace the paraspinal soft-tissue lines. A bulge in the paraspinal soft tissues may indicate:

❏ haemorrhage
❏ tumour
❏ infection and inflammation.

Image periphery
Occasionally, an extraspinal abnormality will be evident, such as a posterior rib fracture or pneumothorax.

Fig. 6.42. AP view of the lumbar spine demonstrating a pathological fracture at T12 secondary to a metastasis. Systematic review of the pedicles demonstrates loss of the left T12 pedicle, which has been destroyed by metastatic infiltration (a). Normal L1 pedicle marked for comparison (b).

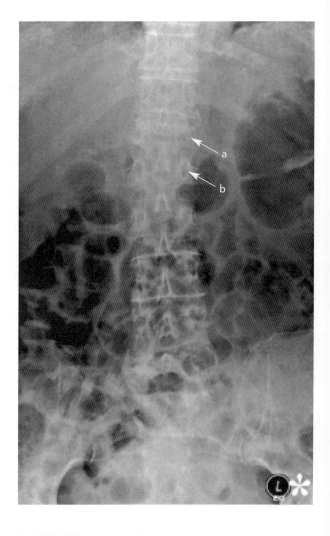

Fig. 6.43. Lateral view of the patient in Fig. 6.42, demonstrating the collapsed T12 vertebra.

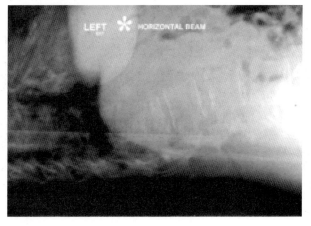

Interpretation Tips

Thoracic and lumbar spine radiograph

- If a destructive spinal abnormality is seen, decide whether it is disc centred (e.g. discitis) or bone based (e.g. metastases) (Fig. 6.44).
- A typical sign of an osteoporotic fracture is a cleavage line through the vertebral body in line with the end-plates.
- Most wedge collapses are osteoporotic, but malignancy should be considered if: there is an associated soft-tissue paraspinal mass, the posterior elements are involved, the collapsed vertebra remains relatively lucent (due to bone destruction), the cortical margins and end-plates are not intact.
- Particularly if neurological compromise is present, have a low threshold for recommending further cross-sectional imaging.

QUICK REFERENCE CHECKLIST

Thoracic and lumbar spine radiograph

Lateral view
- Alignment
- Vertebrae
- Disc spaces

AP view
- Alignment
- Vertebrae
  - Vertebral bodies
  - Pedicles
  - Spinous processes
- Disc spaces
- Paraspinal tissues
- Image periphery

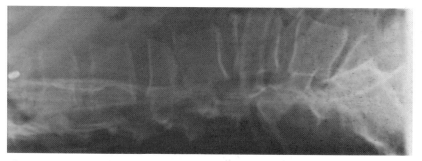

Fig. 6.44. Discitis of the L2–L3 disc. Lateral lumbar spinal radiograph demonstrating destruction of the inferior and superior end-plates of L2 and L3, respectively, due to disc-centred infection.

SPINAL MRI

MRI gives excellent soft-tissue contrast when imaging the spine, unlike CT, which is good at assessing bone detail. A soft-tissue CT algorithm still has an important role to play in those patients who are unable to undergo MR scanning (e.g. claustrophobic patients). Common pathologies imaged with MRI include degenerative disc disease, infection (e.g. discitis), neoplasia and trauma.

Protocol

Sequences

The following scanning protocols are used in our centre.

Sagittal
- ❏ T1
- ❏ T2
- ❏ STIR – optional sequence in those in whom infection, inflammation and tumour are suspected.

Axial
- ❏ T2 – slices of 3–4 mm through region of interest
- ❏ T1 – optional.

Intravenous gadolinium contrast
This contrast agent is used in cases of suspected discitis, the delineation of other inflammatory conditions and for tumours of neural origin. It is also used following disc surgery, to differentiate scarring (diffuse enhancement) from recurrent disc prolapse (either no enhancement or only rim enhancement).

Adequacy

Check that the area of interest is covered and record the vertebral levels encompassed by the scan.

Sagittal sequences

Alignment
- ❏ T1, T2.

As with the plain radiograph of the spine, assess vertebral alignment, checking for forward slip of one vertebral body on another (spondylolisthesis).

Vertebral bodies
- ❏ T1.

Assess vertebral body shape and height (Fig. 6.45). Look at the edges of each vertebral body in turn for irregularity and osteophyte formation.

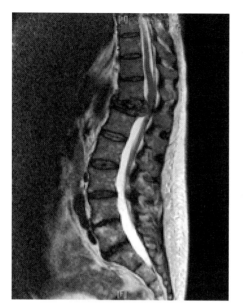

Fig. 6.45. Sagittal T2-weighted MR scan demonstrating metastatic infiltration and collapse of the T12 vertebral body. Note distal spinal cord compression just above the conus.

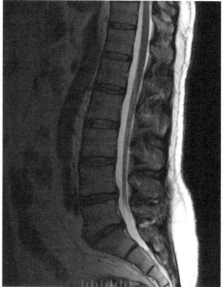

Fig. 6.46. The sagittal T2-weighted view demonstrates dehydrated L4–5 and L5–S1 discs that bulge into the neural canal.

Marrow

Normal marrow is bright on T1, due to a high fat content. Replacement by tumour leads to low T1 signal. STIR suppresses fat signal, but shows oedema as high signal, therefore malignant invasion is dark on T1 and bright on STIR.

Discs

On the T2 sequences assess:

❏ height
❏ hydration (the normal disc centre is bright on T2 due to the high free water content)
❏ degeneration of the disc, which leads to loss of T2 signal from the nucleus pulposus (Figs 6.46 and 6.47)
❏ bulging (if the disc bulges into the spinal canal, note whether there is any impingement on the cord, cauda equina or roots, and check for the 'keyhole sign' on parasagittal sections (due to fat surrounding the emerging nerve root in the exit foramina, which is lost in disc impingement) (Fig. 6.48).

Cord

❏ T2.

Evaluate the size of the cord and the level of the conus, if seen. Check that the cauda equina is not abnormally thickened or nodular. Look for any lesions within,

Fig. 6.47. Axial T2-weighted image of the same patient as in Fig. 6.46 at the L4–5 level demonstrating a right paracentral disc bulge compressing the lateral recess (a).

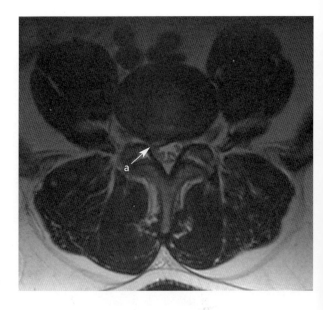

Fig. 6.48. Magnified parasagittal T1-weighted view of the normal 'keyhole'-shaped exit foramina (a), with high-signal fat surrounding the exiting nerve (b).

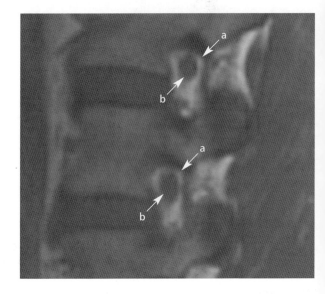

or closely related to, the cord. Try to ascertain the origin of the lesion (Fig. 6.49) and note its signal characteristics (e.g. fluid, solid, mixed etc.).

Any abnormality seen on the sagittal images should be cross-referenced with the corresponding axial sequences.

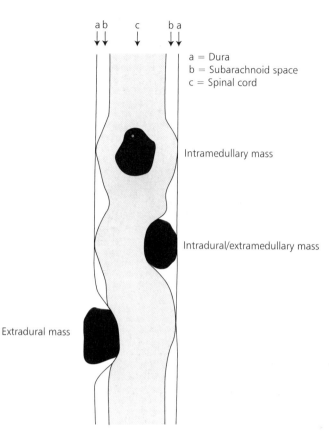

a = Dura
b = Subarachnoid space
c = Spinal cord

Intramedullary mass

Intradural/extramedullary mass

Extradural mass

Fig. 6.49. Spinal masses may leave characteristic impressions on the spinal cord and cerebrospinal fluid, depending on their site of origin.

Axial sequences

Thecal sac
❑ T2.

Look at the shape of the thecal sac. Check that the disc does not bulge into the thecal sac, compressing the cord, cauda equina or nerve roots (see Fig. 6.47).

Nerve roots
This is particularly pertinent within the lumbar spine. Check each nerve root as it exits the patent spinal foramina between the pedicles on the T1 images. Trace each root to the respective plexus. Again, look for disc herniation impinging on nerve roots, which may not have been appreciated on the sagittal images (see Fig 6.47).

Paraspinal soft tissues
Check for paraspinal soft-tissue abnormalities, such as an associated inflammatory soft-tissue mass or an incidental lesion (e.g. renal mass) (Fig. 6.50).

Fig. 6.50. This MR scan was performed for cord compression. The cause for the neural compromise is apparent – metastatic cancer from a left renal primary (a).

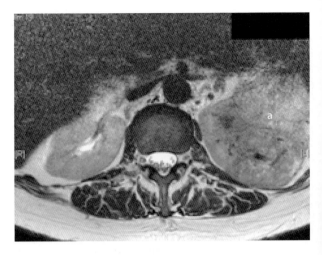

Summary of common conditions

Degenerative/prolapsed disc:

❏ reduced height
❏ dehydrated discs
❏ posterior disc bulge and associated neural compression
❏ free disc fragments.

Neoplasia:
❏ marrow invasion, best seen on T1 and STIR
❏ vertebral body destruction (bulging posterior disc margin)
❏ enhancing soft-tissue mass
❏ neural involvement.

Infection
❏ both high T2 and STIR signal crossing both involved bone and disc
❏ low T1 signal of involved bone and disc

Interpretation Tips

Spine MRI

● T1 sequences are better than T2 sequences at detecting altered marrow signal due to tumour invasion.
● Differentiation between osteophytes and a bulging intervertebral disc can be difficult, especially in the cervical spine.
● Cervical foramina can be difficult to visualize; high-resolution axial T2 sequences may need to be acquired.
● Artefact from the central canal can give false streaks of high signal within the cord, mimicking an intrinsic spinal lesion.
● In the context of trauma, MRI is good at assessing the relationship of retropulsed fragments to the cord.

QUICK REFERENCE CHECKLIST

Spine MRI

Adequacy
Sagittal sequences
● Alignment
● Vertebral bodies
● Marrow
● Discs
● Cord
Axial sequences
● Thecal sac
● Nerve roots
● Paraspinal soft tissue

❏ irregular vertebral cortical margins
❏ associated epidural or paraspinal inflammatory mass
❏ associated with reduced disc space height, unlike neoplasia.

CT MULTITRAUMA

This investigation presents a unique challenge to the unwary, owing to the sheer volume of information requiring interpretation. CT multitrauma scanning is indicated in our centre if:

❏ severe injury is sustained to two, non-related organ systems (i.e. head and spine, chest, abdomen and pelvis or limbs)
❏ trauma was sustained at high velocity (>60 mph)
❏ there is an unknown mechanism of injury, with reduced conscious level (or if this cannot be assessed).

The scanning protocol used in our centre is:

❏ head and neck to the inferior end-plate of T2 – without intravenous contrast
❏ thorax – 30-second delay following 100 ml intravenous contrast
❏ abdomen and pelvis – 70-second delay following intravenous contrast
❏ lower limbs – only if severe injury is apparent
❏ whole-spine small-field sagittal and coronal reconstructions
❏ pelvic three-dimensional bony reformats if pelvic fracture is evident.

Head

Look for both extra- and intracerebral injuries.

Extracerebral injuries include:

❏ fractures of the skull vault, base and facial bones (seen on bone windows)

❏ scalp injury (i.e. lacerations and foreign bodies)
❏ haemorrhage (extradural, subdural or subarachnoid).

Intracerebral injuries include:

❏ diffuse cerebral oedema – swollen brain (effacement of ventricles and basal cisterns, loss of sulci, diffuse low attenuation with loss of grey–white differentiation)
❏ contusions – typically seen within the inferior frontal and anterior temporal lobes, and may be low or high attenuation, depending on whether they contain haemorrhage
❏ diffuse axonal injury – shearing of axons at grey–white interface, which may lead to multifocal punctate haemorrhages. The CT may also appear normal.

Spine

Start with the small-field sagittal, then go on to coronal plain reconstructions of the cervical spine. Look for malalignment of the vertebral bodies and facet joints, and for fractures.

For fractures, check the axial images, carefully correlating abnormalities seen in the sagittal and coronal planes. Repeat the process for the thoracic and lumbar spines.

If a fracture is identified, comment on the degree of displacement, the presence of any retropulsed fragments within the spinal canal and overall spinal stability.

Thorax

Soft-tissue injury

❏ Mediastinal windows

Look for:

❏ aortic injury – check for a dissection flap and aortic wall injury/para-aortic haematoma (commonly seen at the site of the ligamentum arteriosum, just distal to the origin of the left subclavian artery) (Figs 6.51 and 6.52)
❏ mediastinal haematoma
❏ pericardial fluid
❏ chest wall/axilliary haematoma
❏ diaphragmatic injury, which can be difficult to diagnose (the normally well-defined diaphragmatic margin appears indistinct, and is best seen on coronal reconstructions)
❏ position of tubes and lines (e.g. endotracheal tube, central lines, chest drains).

Lung injury

❏ Lung windows.

Look for:

❏ pheumothorax, haemopneumothorax, surgical emphysema

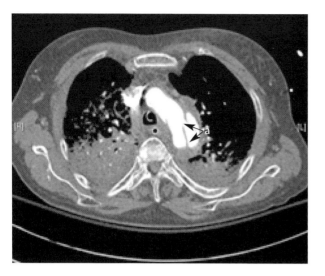

Fig. 6.51. Traumatic aortic dissection (a). In addition, there are bilateral pleural effusions, consolidation and nasogastric and endotracheal tubes.

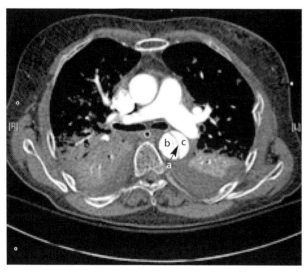

Fig. 6.52. A lower axial section of the same patient as in Fig. 6.51. The dissection flap is clearly seen (a) separating the true (b) and false (c) lumina. Rib fractures are also evident.

❏ pneumomediastinum, which in isolation may indicate bronchial rupture
❏ pulmonary contusions (seen as focal consolidation)
❏ aspirated foreign bodies.

Bone injury

❏ Bone windows.

Look for:

❏ fractures of the ribs (multiple with or without flail segment), sternum and scapulae.

Abdomen and pelvis

Look for:

❏ intra-abdominal free gas (e.g. from gut perforation) (change to lung windows for this)
❏ major vascular injury – follow the aorta, IVC and iliac vessels
❏ free fluid (e.g. haemorrhage)
❏ solid organ injury (low-attenuation laceration with or without subcapsular or extracapsular haematoma) – spleen (Fig. 6.53), liver, kidneys and pancreas (look for active extravasation of contrast and any associated vascular injury)
❏ gut and mesenteric injury – mural thickening and small extraluminal gas bubbles indicate full-thickness gut injury (look for increased attenuation within the mesentery signifying contusion)
❏ bladder injury, indicated by adjacent haematoma or urinoma (delayed scans may well demonstrate a leak, in which case attempt to define whether the leak is intra- or extraperitoneal)
❏ pelvic fracture (bone windows) (Fig. 6.54).

Fig. 6.53. Splenic laceration (a). There is perisplenic haemorrhage (b), as well as perihepatic fluid (c).

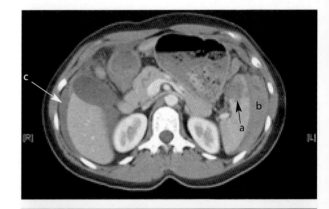

Fig. 6.54. Three-dimensional reconstruction of an 'open book' pelvic injury. There is diastasis of both sacroiliac joints and the pubic symphysis.

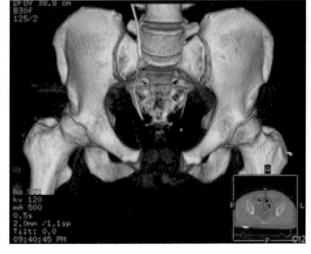

Lower limbs

These are included only if clinically indicated.

Interpretation Tips

CT multitrauma

● Remember the golden rule: never endanger the patient. The primary aim of the multitrauma scan is to identify injury that requires urgent intervention. The patient can always be rescanned at a later point to answer less pressing clinical problems.
● Serious head injury may present with no apparent CT brain abnormality.
● Spinal reconstruction should encompass the occipital condyles, as fractures here are frequently missed.
● Beware of cardiac motion artefact simulating an aortic root dissection. A double aortic root border on both sides of the aorta is likely to be artefactual.
● Common sites for gut injury are those where the bowel is tethered (e.g. duodenal–jejunal flexure).
● Consider delayed urographic phase scans in cases of suspected renal, ureteric or bladder injury.

QUICK REFERENCE CHECKLIST

CT multitrauma

Head
● Extracerebral injury
● Intracerebral injury
Spine
● Alignment
● Fractures
Thorax
● Soft tissues
  – Aorta
  – Mediastinum
  – Pericardial fluid
  – Chest wall/axillae
  – Diaphragm
  – Tubes and lines
● Lungs
  – Pneumothorax, surgical emphysema
  – Pneumomediastinum
  – Contusions
  – Foreign bodies

continued

BONE SCAN

The radionuclide bone scan provides a functional display of skeletal activity. It still plays a pivotal role in identifying metastases from malignant conditions (commonly breast, lung and prostate cancer).

Following injection of tracer (radioactive technetium-labelled diphosphates), static images are acquired with a gamma camera. Tracer uptake reflects areas of osteoblastic activity, but is also dependent on skeletal vascularity. Anterior and posterior whole-body images are acquired approximately 2–4 hours after injection.

Dynamic (on injection) and early blood pool images can be acquired to assess the vascularity of lesions, for example when searching for active infection.

Posterior structures, such as the spine and kidneys, are best appreciated on the posterior view and conversely anterior structures, such as the sternum, are best seen on the anterior view.

The bone scan is very sensitive, but not specific, and interpretation hinges on the recognition of patterns of abnormal tracer uptake. The primary focus of any bone scan should be the identification of potential malignant lesions.

The hallmark of a normal bone scan is symmetry about the midline.

Clinical information

Use this to guide the search for pathology.

Identify areas of increased uptake

Decide whether this is osseous or extra-osseous uptake. Beware of artefactual high uptake, such as extravasation at the injection site.

Patterns of disease

This underpins the interpretation of the bone scan. Try to assess whether lesions are:

❑ multiple or single
❑ symmetrical or asymmetrical
❑ located in the axial or appendicular skeleton.

The following are typical patterns to look for on the bone scan.

Secondary malignancy

Secondary malignancy is characterized by:

❑ multiple lesions, which may spread along bone (Fig. 6.55)
❑ lesions that vary in shape, size and uptake intensity
❑ lesions that have an irregular, asymmetrical distribution
❑ a predilection for the axial skeleton (in only 10% of cases is the appendicular skeleton affected).

Widespread malignancy may cause generalized increased uptake ('superscan').

Degenerative and arthritic changes

These are peri-articular, affecting both sides of the joint, and usually symmetrical (but may vary in intensity between joints). Common sites are hips, knees, lumbar spine, acromioclavicular and sternoclavicular joints.

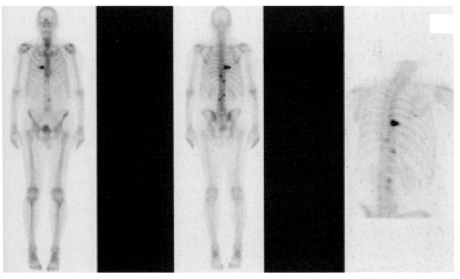

Fig. 6.55. Marked abnormal uptake in the right posterior eighth rib extending along the rib, which also appears expanded. This is highly suggestive of an infiltrating lesion of the bone. While the asymmetrical uptake in the spine is probably due to metastases, bone scan can be non-specific and these areas may represent degenerative disease, and hence correlation with other imaging modalities is helpful.

Trauma

Use clinical information to guide interpretation.

A line of vertical, discrete 'hot spots' on several contiguous ribs is typical of previous rib fractures. Anterior rib ends are also a common site for trauma (Fig. 6.56).

Fig. 6.56. Focal uptake involving three anterior ribs contiguously. The pattern is pathognomonic of fractures.

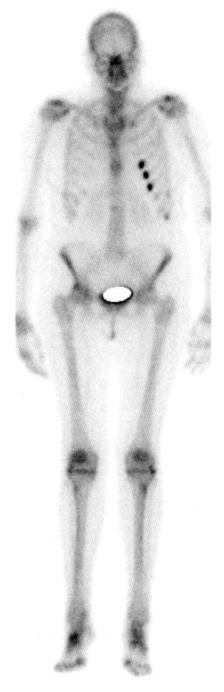

A compressed vertebra that has uniform uptake is typical of osteoporotic collapse.

Infection

Early images show increased vascularity.

Infection shows a predilection for the metaphysis of long bones.

Paget's disease

Paget's disease is more common in elderly people and in 75% of cases is polyostotic. Look for:

- ❏ increased vascularity in early images
- ❏ intense uptake with uniform distribution
- ❏ a predilection for pelvis, lumbar spine, femur, tibia and skull
- ❏ preservation of the normal anatomical configuration (suspect transformation to osteosarcoma when this is not present).

Joint prostheses, infection and loosening

This is a tricky call, but loosening may show as increased uptake at the distal tip of the stem of a hip prosthesis and infection generally manifests as increased uptake around the whole prosthesis

Identify 'cold spots'

Apart from joint prostheses, 'cold spots' or photopenic lesions are usually due to artefacts, such as coins in pockets or jewellery. Previous radiotherapy sites can also demonstrate reduced uptake. Generalized reduced uptake can occur following bisphosphonate therapy. Photopenic lesions are seen in association with aggressive lytic disease, which does not induce an osteoblastic response.

Renal uptake

The tracer is renally excreted, so an approximation of renal size, shape and position can be made. Reduced uptake may indicate renal dysfunction, in which case there may be generalized increased background activity. Increased uptake, usually after chemotherapy, can occur.

There may be such avid skeletal uptake due to widespread metastases that the renal outlines are not seen as there is less tracer to be excreted – the so-called 'superscan'.

Extraosseous uptake

The commonest causes are technical factors, malignancy, myocutaneous conditions, amyloid, infarction, hypercalcaemia, inflammation and chemoradiotherapy.

Previous imaging

Finally, cross-reference the bone scan with previous imaging to aid interpretation.

Interpretation Tips

Bone scan

● An abnormal area can be characterized further by additional oblique or lateral spot views.
● Remember the general rules for malignant deposit: multiple, growing along bones, varying in size, shape and intensity, with an irregular distribution favouring the axial skeleton (see Fig. 6.55).
● Patient rotation can cause apparent increased uptake in the side nearest the detector.
● Identify easy-to-miss 'cold spots' as well as 'hot spots'.
● Do not forget to look for renal and extraosseous uptake.

QUICK REFERENCE CHECKLIST

Bone scan

Clinical information
Identify areas of increased uptake
Patterns of disease
Identify 'cold spots'
Renal uptake
Extraosseous uptake
Compare with previous imaging

VASCULAR RADIOLOGY (7)

LOWER-LIMB ULTRASOUND FOR DEEP-VEIN THROMBOSIS

Ultrasound is a widely available, sensitive and safe way of identifying deep-vein thrombosis (DVT).

Scanning for DVT is often carried out by ultrasonographers or medical physicists; however, it remains an important skill for the radiology trainee to possess.

Scanning protocol

Vessels to be imaged:

❏ common femoral vein
❏ proximal profunda femoris vein
❏ superficial femoral vein
❏ popliteal vein.

Scanning of the calf veins, iliac veins and IVC may also be indicated.

The thigh veins can be scanned with the patient upright, tilted or supine, with the leg externally rotated. The popliteal vein can be imaged with patients standing or lying on their side, or sat on the edge of the bed with their foot supported on a chair. Start with a high-frequency linear probe, although a curvilinear transducer may be needed for larger patients or deeper veins.

Start in the groin, applying light pressure to the common femoral vein until the walls appose. Move down the leg, repeating this process in both the longitudinal and the transverse planes. Use both colour and spectral Doppler to confirm or refute the presence of a thrombus (see below). It may be helpful to support the thigh with the other hand, to aid compression.

There is some conjecture as to whether the calf veins should be scanned routinely, owing to the lower risk of pulmonary thromboembolism and the higher level of inherent scanning inaccuracy in inexperienced hands. Suffice it to say scanning technique is the same as for above the knee. Bear in mind that the deep veins of the calf are paired with their respective artery.

It is important to be familiar with the normal anatomy and ultrasound appearances of the deep leg veins, before attempting to identify the signs of thrombus.

Normal findings

Veins appear:

❏ to be thin walled and larger than the corresponding artery
❏ to be compressible with transducer pressure
❏ to have a smooth anechoic internal lumen
❏ to have a slow phasic flow with respiration on spectral Doppler
❏ to show cessation of flow and vein distension with Valsalva manoeuvre.

On colour Doppler, flow fills the entire lumen and squeezing the calf increases colour flow.

Figs 7.1 and 7.2 show the normal venous appearances.

Fig. 7.1. Longitudinal view of a normal common femoral vein before compression.

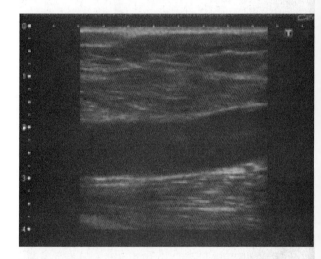

Fig. 7.2. Longitudinal view of a normal common femoral vein after compression.

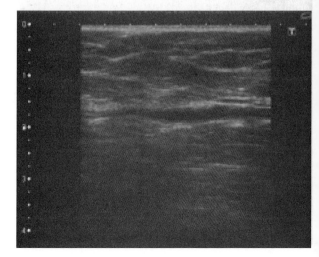

Abnormal findings

Direct evidence of thrombus

Look for:

❏ inability to compress the vein with transducer pressure

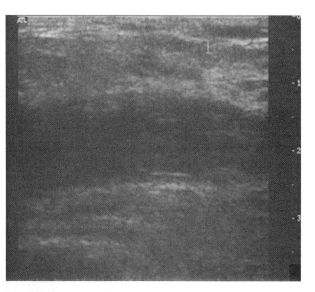

Fig. 7.3. Longitudinal view of the common femoral vein, demonstrating reflective, intraluminal thrombus.

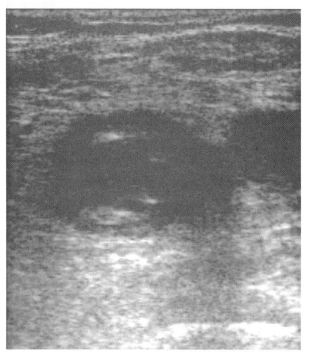

Fig. 7.4. Transverse views of the common femoral vein, demonstrating reflective, intraluminal thrombus.

❏ intraluminal echogenic thrombus (acute clot may be poorly echogenic)
❏ increased luminal diameter in acute thrombus, reduced diameter in chronic thrombus
❏ vein wall thickening
❏ absent flow in occlusive thrombus.

Indirect evidence of thrombus

Look for:

❏ loss of phasic flow with respiration or Valsalva manoeuvre, which suggests proximal venous obstruction
❏ loss of venous distension on Valsalva manoeuvre
❏ minimal increase in flow on squeezing the calf
❏ increased flow in superficial veins and deep collaterals.

Figs 7.3 and 7.4 show venous thrombosis.

Interpretation Tips

Lower-limb ultrasound for deep-vein thrombosis

● Always scan the contralateral leg, because there is a risk of contralateral DVT.
● DVT may be associated with intra-abdominal pathology and an abdominal and pelvic ultrasound scan is often indicated to identify patent iliac vessels and IVC. In addition, search for pelvic/abdominal mass lesions, particularly pelvic lymphadenopathy compressing the iliac vessels, to explain DVT.
● If ultrasound fails to detect above-knee thrombus, and a high clinical probability of DVT remains, it is prudent to rescan the affected limb after one week. It is worth checking the hospital's guidelines on DVT scanning.
● It is important to alert the clinicians if echogenic material is identified floating within the vein, especially within the common femoral and iliac veins, signifying non-adherent thrombus with an inherently higher risk of thromboembolism.
● Squeezing the calf to augment venous flow proximally can provide false reassurance of patency in the presence of non-occlusive thrombus and collateral venous supply. Beware of the small, but important, risk of causing embolism with over-enthusiastic calf squeezing.
● Become familiar with the common appearances of the unilateral swollen limb, including Baker's cyst, deep haematoma and cellulitis.
● Venous duplication is common (up to 20% of superficial femoral veins and 35% of popliteal veins) and may confuse the inexperienced.

Lower-limb ultrasound for deep-vein thrombosis

Vessels to be imaged:
- common femoral vein
- proximal profunda femoris vein
- superficial femoral vein
- popliteal vein
- calf veins, iliac veins and IVC dictated by clinical need.

Remember the direct and indirect signs of thrombus.

TIPS ON PAEDIATRIC INTERPRETATION

In addition to the everyday issues of interpreting imaging studies in adults, under-taking and reporting radiology in children presents several unique challenges:

❏ When performing studies using ionizing radiation, be aware that children are significantly more susceptible to the damaging effects of radiation, and so their exposure must be minimized.
❏ Children are much less likely than adults to cooperate, and specific techniques need to be employed to engage their involvement and secure a diagnostic study.
❏ It is necessary to be conversant with developmental changes and the varying appearances of the growing patient.
❏ It is necessary to have knowledge of the discrete pathologies and diseases that affect children in order to correctly interpret an image.

Because of the issues with ionizing radiation, paediatric imaging places a greater reliance on plain films and ultrasound. It is particularly important to be familiar with the range of normal appearances for age and size, particularly in the most com-monly performed investigations, as described below.

PLAIN FILMS

General issues with plain film interpretation

Artefacts can make a significant contribution to the appearance of the film, partic-ularly in pre-term infants.

Look for mattress artefact (mottled shadowing that mimics the ground-glass pat-tern of surfactant deficiency disorder).

Be aware that ECG and other monitors can cover a significant proportion of the field of view and can mask important pathology.

Beware of 'incubator hole' artefact, which can mimic a loculated pneumothorax or pneumoperitoneum.

Chest radiograph

First assess the technical adequacy of the film:

❏ Check for rotation. Are the medial ends of the clavicles equidistant from the midline? Are the ribs symmetrical? The patient will be rotated *towards* the side

Fig. 8.1. Infant markedly rotated to the right causing distortion of mediastinum with apparent dextrocardia and asymmetrical lungs.

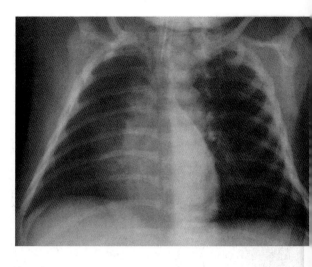

where the posterior ribs are elongated and the anterior ribs appear foreshortened (Fig. 8.1).

❏ Check for inspiratory effort: counting ribs visible above the diaphragm is useful but does not take the place of familiarity with the appearance of a well-inspired exposure at different ages.

❏ Check for lordosis/kyphosis. If the patient is kyphotic, not only may the chin obscure the upper zones, but the upper lobes become aligned parallel to, rather than at right angles to, the beam, and upper-lobe pathology may be completely obscured. Remember that a lordotic film can be useful for revealing middle-lobe pathology.

❏ Become familiar with the varied appearance of the thymus. This is a very fluid structure which can occupy a position anywhere between the neck and the diaphragm. It may have an undulating border or its lower margin may mimic the horizontal fissure. Remember that the thymus responds rapidly to stress such as infection, causing it to involute, and that rebound thymic hyperplasia can occur when the stress is relieved, which can be misinterpreted as a mediastinal mass if the chest radiograph is viewed out of clinical context.

Both because infants tend to be imaged supine and because of the contribution of the thymus, the allowable cardiothoracic ratio is up to 60% rather than 50%.

Make a note of the position of all lines, catheters and other support tubes: endotracheal tube malposition is the commonest cause of lobar or lung collapse in infants (Fig. 8.2).

Right upper-lobe collapse frequently mimics consolidation, as the lobe does not always collapse towards the mediastinum, but instead the volume loss is predominantly in the AP plane. Consequently, there may be no appreciable elevation of the horizontal fissure and increased lung density may be the only sign.

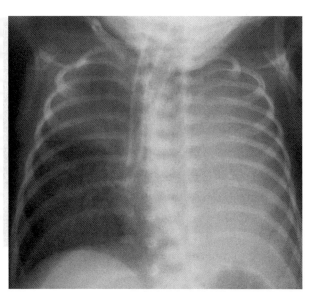

Fig. 8.2. Endotracheal tube in right bronchus intermedius, causing complete collapse of the left lung and partial collapse of the right upper lobe.

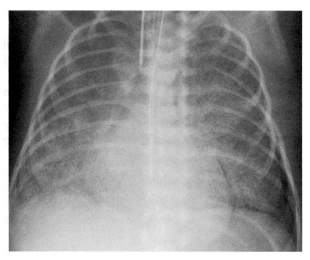

Fig. 8.3. Subtle left pneumothorax: note the thin translucent crescents outlining the left heart border and just above the left hemidiaphragm.

The patterns of pneumothorax in infants and young children also differ from those seen in adults. Rather than seeing the lung edge towards the apex with an absence of lung markings superiorly, the lung margin may parallel the lateral border of the thoracic cage in the case of a lamellar pneumothorax. An anterior pneumothorax may present as a subtle increase in transradiancy of the affected hemithorax, but remember that any rotation of the patient can cause a similar discrepancy in transradiancy of the hemithoraces.

Finally, pleural air commonly collects in a subpulmonary location and may appear as a translucent crescent paralleling the diaphragm or may mimic subpulmonary cysts (Fig. 8.3).

Abdominal radiograph

Bowel

The colon in infants and young children does not demonstrate a haustral pattern and bowel morphology cannot generally be used to differentiate between large and small bowel in infants. The position of the gas-filled loops of bowel may help, the colon being generally more peripherally sited, but the sigmoid colon is often redundant in young children and can extend into the right upper quadrant. The caecum also not infrequently appears to lie higher than expected in infants. Be careful, therefore, when trying to determine the level of obstruction in an infant: unless the valvulae conniventes can clearly be seen, do not assume that the small bowel is being seen (Fig. 8.4).

The best indicator of the level of obstruction is the number of gas-filled loops present.

Calcification

Calcification is far more likely to be pathological when seen on a child's abdominal film. Causes of calcification in infants include meconium peritonitis and congenital infection.

Fig. 8.4. Obstruction of the small bowel. The peripheral distribution suggests that the dilated bowel represents colon, but valvulae conniventes are clearly visible in the right upper quadrant, confirming that this is ileum.

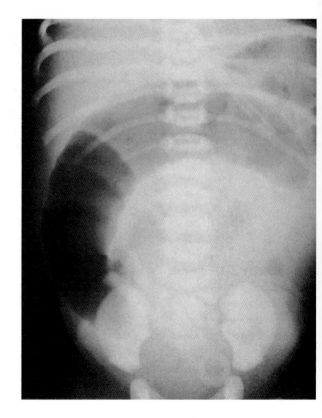

In older children with abdominal pain, look for an appendicolith and remember that renal stones have become significantly more prevalent in the paediatric population since the early 1990s.

Extremity radiographs

When interpreting appendicular skeletal images in children, it is important to remember the following:

❏ Multiple, fragmented and accessory ossification centres may be mistaken for fractures. When reporting paediatric skeletal radiographs, it is helpful to have a textbook at hand illustrating normal anatomical variants.
❏ Paediatric fractures may involve the growth plate and these can result in growth disturbance, so it is important to identify them and make this clear in the report. The Salter–Harris classification is the most commonly used method of describing epiphyseal fractures (Fig. 8.5).
❏ Knowledge of the sequence in which ossification centres are expected to appear is helpful both in determining skeletal maturity and in assessing fractures involving unossified cartilage.
❏ The distal femoral and proximal tibial ossification centres should be present by 36 weeks of gestation.

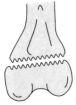

Salter–Harris I
Fracture line runs through the physis

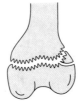

Salter–Harris II
Fracture line passes through a corner of the metaphysis, then along the physis

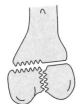

Salter–Harris III
Fracture line passes through a corner of the epiphysis, then along the physis

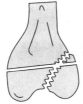

Salter–Harris IV
Fracture line runs through metaphysis, physis and epiphysis

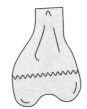

Salter–Harris V
Compression of the physis with no visible fracture line

Fig. 8.5. The Salter–Harris classification of epiphyseal fractures.

❑ The order of appearance of centres at the elbow is usually capitellum–radial head–internal epicondyle–trochlea–olecranon–external epicondyle.

ULTRASOUND

When undertaking paediatric ultrasound, it is important to adjust scanning parameters to suit the young patient.

❑ An intermediate-frequency (5–7.5 MHz) curvilinear probe is used most commonly, selecting paediatric set-ups that are available on all modern machines.
❑ Optimize resolution by reducing depth of field to the shallowest possible that still includes the area of interest and only then utilizing zoom.
❑ Even though it may not be possible to include the whole organ or structure, supplementing curvilinear scanning by using a linear high-frequency (7.5–12 MHz) probe can be very useful for assessing texture, flow and fine detail.

Renal ultrasound

This is the most commonly undertaken paediatric ultrasound examination. Get into the habit of always starting by scanning the bladder: this is crucial in babies, who often void as soon as a probe is put on their abdomen.

Assess bladder wall thickness (should be no more than 3 mm in the distended bladder), bladder shape, any intravesical lesions – cystic (e.g. ureterocoele) or solid (e.g. bladder tumour) – and the retrovesical region. Record the diameter of any visible ureter.

Scan the kidneys with the patient in the supine/supine oblique position: assess echotexture relative to liver/spleen and identify any dilatation of the collecting system. If the upper ureter is dilated, it is easier to follow it down with the patient in the supine position.

Scan the kidneys in longitudinal and transverse planes with the patient in the prone position. Measure maximal longitudinal diameter and assess pelvicalyceal dilatation. Document any calyceal distension even if the renal pelvis is not enlarged. Measure the diameter of the renal pelvis in the AP plane (not coronal).

Assess the renal outline for focal defects (e.g. renal scars) and look for focal intrarenal lesions (e.g. duplication, cysts, stones, masses) (Fig. 8.6).

Dilated collecting systems may be developmental, or due to reflux or obstruction. Look for ureteric jets in the bladder using colour Doppler. Assess how far distal the collecting system is dilated and document whether the dilatation is unilateral or bilateral. Remember that dilated collecting systems in the male infant may indicate posterior urethral valves: a bladder wall thickness of 4 mm or above should be considered due to posterior urethral valves until proven otherwise.

It is normal for the echogenicity of the renal cortex to be greater than that of adjacent liver parenchyma for the first 3 months of life, with absence of the expected

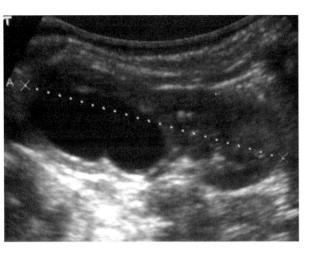

Fig. 8.6. Renal ultrasound showing a duplex kidney with dilated upper moiety.

cortico-medullary differentiation. This makes the renal pyramids stand out as hypo-echoic triangles, which can be misinterpreted as hydronephrosis.

In renal agenesis, the adrenal glands can appear particularly prominent and their multilayered appearance can occasionally mimic a dysplastic kidney.

General abdominopelvic ultrasound

In the neonate, the uterus is frequently stimulated by maternal hormones and may be prominent.

Hypertrophic pyloric stenosis

Start by using the linear probe transversely in the epigastrium and move inferiorly using the liver as a window until the stomach outlet is identified. The pyloric canal should measure no more than 14 mm in length and individual muscle wall thickness should be less than 2.5 mm. Measurements greater than these are indicative of hypertrophic pyloric stenosis.

Suspected intussusception

Start with a curvilinear probe, as it is easier to become properly orientated: an intussusception will be clearly identifiable at frequencies of 5–7 MHz. Document any free fluid and any fluid trapped in the intussusception, together with any potential lead point, such as prominent lymph nodes.

Suspected testicular torsion

Testicular blood flow remains unreliable in the assessment of suspected testicular torsion in young boys and must be interpreted with caution.

CT

Technique

Ideally, scanning parameters should be adjusted for patient size and for the area under review: mA and kV should be just sufficient to achieve a diagnostic study, which frequently means that the images are not 'pretty' but nevertheless allow a diagnosis to be confidently made.

When imaging the chest, very low mA and kV can be successfully used if mediastinal detail is not required, owing to the inherent contrast provided between aerated lungs and the interstitium.

High-resolution lung scanning can nowadays be more reliably achieved in younger patients, while the speed of multislice scanning has greatly reduced the need for sedation in young patients.

Pre-contrast imaging is only rarely necessary: post-contrast scans alone are adequate for diagnosis and this halves patient dose. Similarly, multiphase liver imaging is undertaken in only the assessment of hepatic malignancy.

Scanning delay after contrast administration is generally much less than in adults and should take into account a faster heart rate and shorter vascular travelling distance.

Interpretation

When assessing the mediastinum, remember the thymus and its variability: it is normal for children up to the age of 5 years to have a convex thymic border.

Lung nodules are more likely to be pathological in children, even when solitary.

The paucity of intra-abdominal fat in children makes the interpretation of abdominal CT problematic; oral contrast is all the more important.

FLUOROSCOPY

Studies of the upper gastrointestinal tract

These usually employ a single-contrast technique, as fine mucosal detail is not generally necessary in infants and young children. In barium swallows look for:

❑ laryngeal penetration (is the swallow safe?)
❑ extrinsic compression of the oesophagus (e.g. aberrant vessels, vascular rings)
❑ strictures (usually due to reflux or occasionally postoperative)
❑ dysmotility, especially in the presence of known congenital abnormality, such as previous tracheo-oesophageal fistula
❑ hiatus hernia.

In barium meals also look for:

❏ gastric lie (is the stomach more horizontal than usual, and does the pylorus lie lower than the gastro-oesophageal junction?)
❏ rate of gastric emptying
❏ the position of the duodenojejunal flexure, which should lie on or to the left of the left spinal pedicle in a non-rotated AP projection.

Micturating cystourethrography

This examination is most frequently undertaken to assess the presence of reflux and any underlying developmental anomaly. It is vital to minimize dose to the pelvis, and hence immaculate technique is required.

Filling views of the bladder should be assessed for shape and any intravesical lesion. Ureteroceles may become less apparent as the bladder becomes fuller. Bladder trabeculation implies an outlet obstruction or neuropathy.

Voiding views, particularly in males, should be obtained with the catheter removed. Assess the entire length of the urethra, as 5% of pathology lies in the anterior third. Look for any calibre change that might indicate an obstruction such as posterior urethral valves, strictures or diverticula. A post-void cross-kidney view must be obtained to exclude subtle reflux missed during voiding. The report should include an indication of the degree of any reflux seen.

MRI

Paediatric MRI largely lies outside the scope of this text, but several basic principles are worth stating:

❏ With younger patients, it is important to start with the sequence that is most likely to yield a diagnosis, rather than sticking rigidly to a protocol, as it is not possible to tell how long a child will tolerate being in the scanner.
❏ For musculoskeletal MRI, always review any plain films before attempting to interpret the scan. This will avoid the embarrassment of misdiagnosing a developmental variant as pathology.
❏ Knowing how marrow signal return changes with age is vital, particularly when reviewing scans on patients with known or suspected malignancy.

QUICK REFERENCE CHECKLIST

Paediatric interpretation

● Minimize patient exposure to radiation.
● Know the normal developmental variants.
● Check technical aspects of the study before assessing images for pathology.

FURTHER READING

General

Dahnert W. *Radiology Review Manual*. Philadelphia: Lippincott, Williams & Wilkins, 2007.

Howling SJ, Jenkins P, Grundy A, Wasan R. *Radiology for MRCP 2*. Knutsford: PasTest, 2003.

Neuroradiology

Carter RMS, Pretorius RM. The use of CT and MR in the characterization of intra-cranial mass lesions. *Imaging* 2007; **19**: 173–84.

Harden SP, Dey C, Gawne Cain ML. Cranial CT of the unconscious adult patient. *Clin Radiol* 2007; **62**: 404–15.

Srinivasan A, Goyal M, Al Azri F, Lum C. State-of-the-art imaging of acute stroke. *Radiographics* 2006; **26**(suppl 1): S75–95.

Head and neck radiology

Ahuja AT, Evans RM. *Practical Head and Neck Ultrasound*. Cambridge: Greenwich Medical Media, 2000.

Ahuja AT, Yuen HY, Wong KT, Yue V, van Hasselt AC. Computed tomography imaging of the temporal bone – normal anatomy. *Clin Radiol* 2003; **58**: 681–6.

Blunt DM. Non-laryngeal squamous cell carcinoma of the upper aerodigestive tract. *Imaging* 2003; **15**: 95–100.

Brant WE, Helms CA. *Fundamentals of Diagnostic Radiology*. Philadelphia: Lippincott, Williams & Wilkins, 2007.

Dubrulle F, Souillard R, Hermans R. Extension patterns of nasopharyngeal carcinoma. *Eur Radiol* 2007; **17**: 2622–30.

Siddiqui A, Connor SEJ. Imaging the pharynx and larynx. *Imaging* 2007; **19**: 83–103.

Chest radiology

Corne J, Carroll M, Delany D, Brown I. *Chest X-Ray Made Easy*, 2nd edn. London: Churchill Livingstone, 2002.

Elsenhuber E. The tree-in-bud sign. *Radiology* 2002; **222**: 771–2.

Tuddenham WJ. Glossary of terms for thoracic radiology: recommendations of the Nomenclature Committee of the Fleischner Society. *Am J Roentgenol* 1984; **143**: 509–17.

Ziessman HA, O'Malley JP, Thrall JH. *Nuclear Medicine: The Requisites*, 3rd edn. London: Elsevier/Mosby, 2006.

Breast radiology

Brant WE, Helms CA. *Fundamentals of Diagnostic Radiology*. Philadelphia: Lippincott, Williams & Wilkins, 2007.
Dahnert W. *Radiology Review Manual*. Philadelphia: Lippincott, Williams & Wilkins, 2007.

Abdominal radiology

Bates JA. *Abdominal Ultrasound: How, Why and When*. London: Elsevier, 2004.
Breen DJ, Rutherford EE, Stedman B, Lee-Elliott C, Hacking CN. Intrahepatic arterioportal shunting and anomalous venous drainage: understanding the CT features in the liver. *Eur Radiol* 2004; **14**: 2249–60.
Cosgrove D, ed. *Clinical Ultrasound: Abdominal and General Ultrasound*. London: Churchill Livingstone, 2000.
Dogra VS, Gottlieb RH, Oka M, Rubens DJ. Sonography of the scrotum. *Radiology* 2003; **227**: 18–36.
Federle MP. CT of the acute (emergency) abdomen. *Eur Radiol* 2005; **15** (suppl):D100–4
Hofer M. *Ultrasound Teaching Manual*. New York: Thième, 2005.
Howlett DC, Marchbank NDP, Sallomi DF. Ultrasound of the testis – pictorial review. *Clin Radiol* 2000; **55**: 595–601.
Maglinte DD, Balthazar EJ, Kelvin FM, Megibow AJ. The role of radiology in the diagnosis of small bowel obstruction. *Am J Roentgenol* 1997; **168**: 1171–80.
Martyin L, Wastie ML, Rockall A. *Diagnostic Imaging*, 5th edn. Oxford: Blackwell Science, 2004.
Middleton WD, Kurtz AB, Hertzberg BS. *Ultrasound: The Requisites*. St Louis, MI: Mosby, 2004.
Mindelzun RE, Jeffrey RB Jr, Lane MJ, Silverman PM. The misty mesentery on CT: differential diagnosis. *Am J Roentgenol* 1996; **167**: 61–5.
Nicholson DA, Driscoll PA. ABC of emergency radiology. The abdomen – 1. *BMJ* 1993; **307**: 1342–6.
Nicholson DA, Driscoll PA. ABC of emergency radiology. The abdomen – 2. *BMJ* 1993; **307**: 1410–14.
Pandharipande PV, Krinsky GA, Rusinek H, Lee VS. Perfusion imaging of the liver: current challenges and future goals. *Radiology* 2005; **234**: 661–73.
Siewert B, Raptopoulos V. CT of the acute abdomen: findings and impact on diagnosis and treatment. *Am J Roentgenol* 1994; **163**: 1317–24.

Musculoskeletal radiology

Aliabadi P, Tumeh SS, Weissman BN, McNeil BJ. Cemented total hip prosthesis: radiographic and scintigraphic evaluation. *Radiology* 1989; **173**: 203–6.

Barron D. Imaging trauma of the appendicular skeleton. *Imaging* 2007; **19**: 323–5.

Chan O. *ABC of Emergency Radiology*. London: BMJ Books (Blackwell Publishing), 2007.

Domb BG, Tyler W, Ellis S, McCarthy E. Radiographic evaluation of pathological bone lesions: current spectrum of disease and approach to diagnosis. *J Bone Joint Surg Am* 2004; **86**: 84–90.

Gibbs CP, Weber K, Scarborough MT. Malignant bone tumors. *J Bone Joint Surg Am* 2001; **83A**: 1728–45.

Ostlere S. Imaging the ankle. *Imaging* 2007; **19**: 269–98.

Raby N, Berman L, de Lacey G. *Accident and Emergency Radiology: A Survival Guide*. Oxford: Saunders/Elsevier, 2005.

Stoller DW, ed. *Magnetic Resonance Imaging: MRI in Orthopaedics and Rheumatology*. Philadelphia: Lippincott, 1989.

Taljanovic MS, Jones MD, Hunter TB, Benjamin JB, Ruth JT, Brown AW, Sheppard JE. Joint arthroplasties and prostheses. *Radiographics* 2003; **23**: 1295–314.

Watt I. Basic differential diagnosis of arthritis. *Eur Radiol* 1997; **7**: 344–51.

Weismann BN. Imaging of total hip replacement. *Radiology* 1997; **202**: 611–23.

Vascular radiology

Clough A. *Making Sense of Vascular Ultrasound: A Hands-On Guide*. London: Arnold, 2004.

Kaufman JA, Lee MJ. *Vascular and Interventional Radiology: The Requisites*. London: Mosby, 2003.

Paediatric radiology

Keats TE, Anderson MW. *Atlas of Normal Roentgen Variants That May Simulate Disease*, 7th edn. London: Mosby, 2001.

INDEX

Page references to figures, tables and text boxes are shown in *italics*. Page references to "Quick Reference Checklists" and "Interpretation Tips" are shown in **bold**.

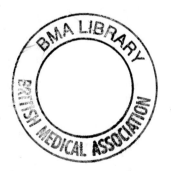